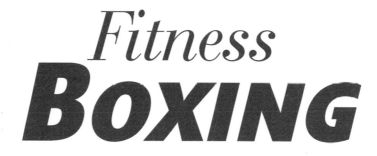

Fitness
BOXING

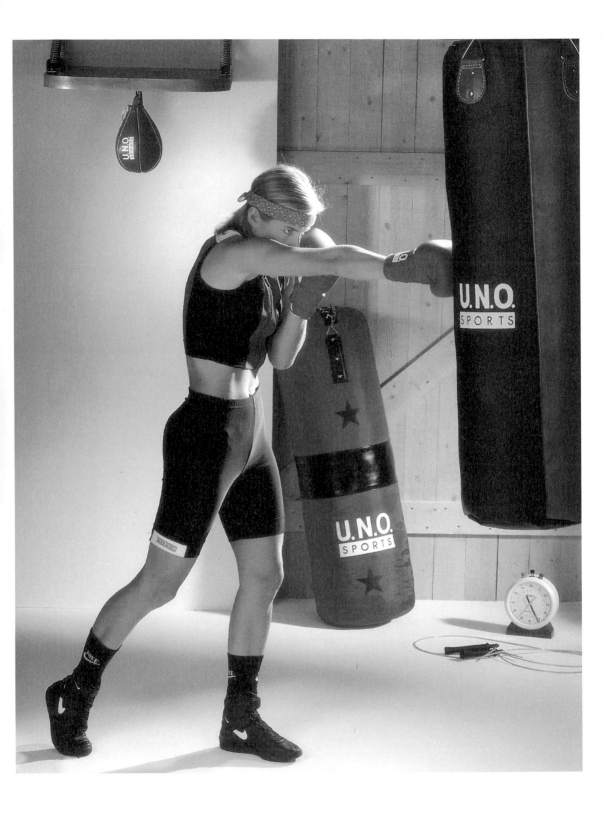

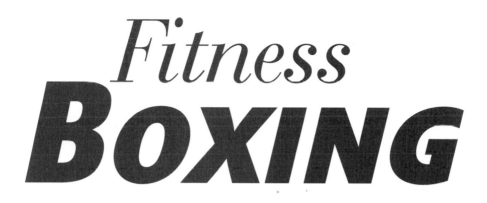

Fitness BOXING

Frank Kurzel & Peter Wastl

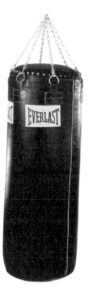

Sterling Publishing Co., Inc.
New York

796.83
Kur

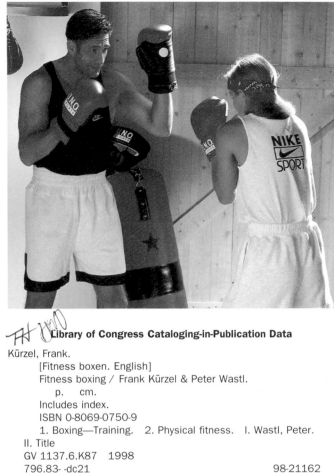

Library of Congress Cataloging-in-Publication Data

Kürzel, Frank.
   [Fitness boxen. English]
   Fitness boxing / Frank Kürzel & Peter Wastl.
      p.   cm.
   Includes index.
   ISBN 0-8069-0750-9
   1. Boxing—Training.   2. Physical fitness.   I. Wastl, Peter.
  II. Title
  GV 1137.6.K87   1998
  796.83- -dc21   98-21162
                             CIP

Photo Credits on page 93

10 9 8 7 6 5 4 3 2 1

Published by Sterling Publishing Company, Inc.
387 Park Avenue South, New York, N.Y. 10016
Originally published in German under the title *Fitness Boxen* and
  copyright © 1997 by FALKEN Verlag, Niederhausen/Ts.
English translation © 1998 by Published by Sterling Publishing Co., Inc.
Distributed in Canada by Sterling Publishing
℅ Canadian Manda Group, One Atlantic Avenue, Suite 105
Toronto, Ontario, Canada M6K 3E7
Distributed in Great Britain and Europe by Cassell PLC
Wellington House, 125 Strand, London WC2R 0BB, England
Distributed in Australia by Capricorn Link (Australia) Pty Ltd.
P.O. Box 6651, Baulkham Hills, Business Centre, NSW 2153, Australia

Sterling ISBN 0-8069-0750-9

CONTENTS

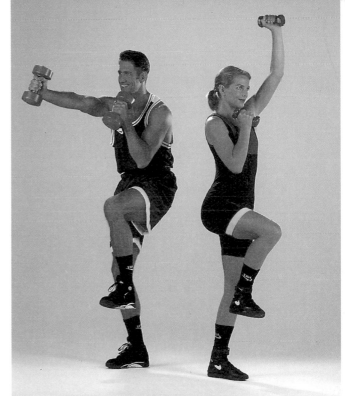

PREFACE

Today fitness boxing is recognized as a significant, health-promoting exercise program that provides a versatile and complete workout. Fitness boxing is a variation of actual boxing in which real punches are never exchanged at any time. The training consists primarily of exercises done with and without exercise equipment, as well as work on the speed and heavy bags, and training using padded gloves. The workout and punching exercises improve basic motor skills, strength, endurance, speed, and coordination, and are excellent for reducing aggression and increasing concentration. This training also increases self-confidence and emotional well-being. And it does this better than almost any other type of sport or exercise.

Benefits from fitness boxing include well-developed muscle strength, increased stamina, and improvement to concentration and reflexes. These benefits make it easier to deal with everyday stress. Improvement to concentration and reflexes is useful not only in the working environment, but also when pursuing recreational activities.

This book describes a training program that is appropriate for men and women yet adaptable to individual abilities, useful for boxers and amateur athletes, and an ideal way to train at home. Included is information about how fitness boxing relates to basic exercise principles, tips about proper clothing and equipment, and seven specially chosen training programs. More than 60 exercises deal with stretching, and improving strength, stamina, coordination, and response time. In addition, we have also included tips for performing proper boxing techniques in front of a mirror, practicing on heavy and speed bags, and training with a partner with and without contact.

Have fun with fitness boxing!

Frank Kürzel
Dr. Peter Wastl

WHAT IS FITNESS BOXING?

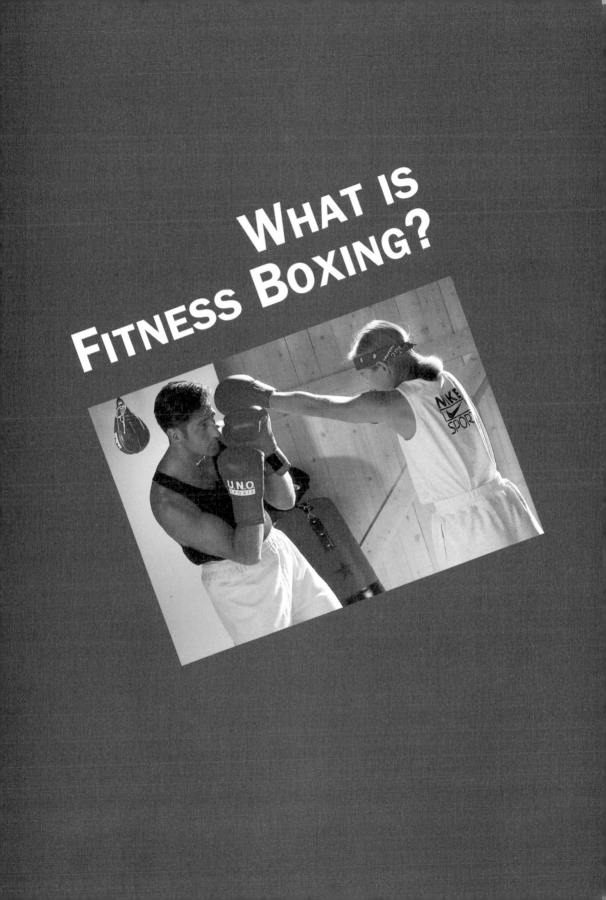

ORIGIN AND DEVELOPMENT

Boxing, the sport of fighting with your fists, has been known as long as 5,000 years, particularly in China, Egypt, and Indonesia. This makes it one of the oldest sports in the world.

During the 7th and 8th centuries B.C., boxing played a considerable role in Greece in the fitness training of the young people, and was considered necessary training for people in the political-military arena. This was because boxing as a sport supported the ideal image that Greeks had of the human body. They knew that its powerful and precise movements shaped the total body and thereby promoted quickness and coordination. To reduce the impact of the punches, they protected their hands with leather bandages and provided protection for the head.

This version of fist-fighting later degenerated to exhibition fights that were meant to quench the masses' desire for violence. Bandages, leather strips and knuckle-dusters were modified to such an extent that the effects of the hitting were emphasized.

The Romans used boxing as part of their military training and competitions. Fights between professional boxers and gladiators were held in front of an audience.

Boxing as an independent competitive sport disappeared from Europe for the next thousand years. Not until the end of the Middle Ages did boxing reappear in the form of "freestyle wrestling," and was then taught in fencing schools.

Modern boxing as we know it today did not surface until the 17th century in England. At the beginning of the 18th century, it became better known as Exhibition Fights, carried out between professional fencers and boxers. For the first time, basic rules were established and the first textbooks were published. But it was not until the 19th century that this form of boxing developed into a competitive sport in the Anglo-Saxon countries. Clubs and associations were formed, and explicit rules and weight classes were established. The obligatory use of boxing gloves was instituted, as were the rounds system and time limitations. Existing rules for professional and amateur boxing continued to be improved to promote correct techniques and to prevent uncontrolled hitting.

The Olympic games provided an additional impetus to the sport of boxing. It was during the Olympic Games in St. Louis in 1904 that boxing competitions were held for the first time. With short interruptions, the sport of boxing since 1920 has been a constant in the Olympics.

Since a professional boxing match consists of a maximum of 12 rounds, each lasting three minutes with one minute pause in between,

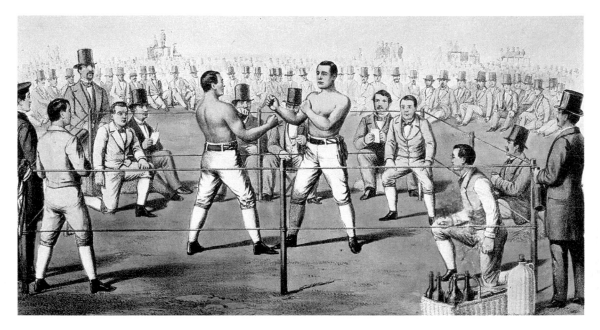

Boxing match with bare fists around 1700.

you might well understand the physical and psychological stamina an athlete needs to sustain such a feat. Developing such stamina requires the boxer to undergo an extensive and intense training program. Specific exercises also train reaction and concentration.

The potential benefits of boxing-specific exercises have been part of fitness training as early as the late 1980s, particularly in America. Sports scientists and physicians have discovered that a fitness-oriented boxing training is one of the best forms of exercises because it conditions the total body.

Boxing from the distant past to today

3rd century B.C.	Evidence of fist-fighting competition in civilized cultures of Egypt, China and Indonesia.
688 B.C.	For the first time, boxing competitions are held in the Olympic Games.
1681	Boxing resurfaces in England after having totally disappeared in Europe during the Middle Ages.
1700	James Figg establishes the first modern rules in boxing and gives it new life. Fighting took place without gloves and lasted until one of the competitors was unable to continue, often lasting as long as 30-60 rounds.
1719	James Figg opens the first boxing school in Tottenham, England.
1743	Jack Broughton reinterprets boxing rules. They remain in use for almost 100 years.
1747	John Godfrey publishes the first textbook on boxing.
1838	"Rules for the Ring in London" are drawn up. A round is terminated when the opponent is down.
1867	A Scottish aristocrat, John Sholto Douglas, 8th Marquis of Queensberry, publishes what is still the basic framework governing boxing with gloves, known as the Queensberry Rules. They consist of 12 rules (among others, the three-minute limit for each round, one-minute break between each, and the use of padded boxing gloves) that were meant, most of all, to stop the brutal excesses of boxing, like leg hooking, throwing the opponent on the ground, and strangling.

1882	First official world competition of professional boxing.
1904	Boxing becomes an Olympic sport at the 3rd modern Olympic games in St. Louis.
1920	First official German championship of amateur boxers in Berlin.
1930	Max Schmeling wins the World Championship of professional boxers in heavyweight division against Jack Sharkey (United States), who was disqualified because of hitting below the belt.
1937-1949	Joe Louis (The Brown Bomber) wins the World Championship in the heavyweight division, and remains champion for almost 12 years, defending his title successfully 25 times.
1964	Muhammad Ali (originally Cassius Clay) wins the World Championship in the heavyweight division of professional boxing and reclaims his title twice, in 1974 and 1978.
1972 -1980	The Cuban heavyweight champion Teofilo Stevenson wins the Olympic gold medal three times in a row.
1975	First official World Championship of amateur boxing.
1988	Henry Maske wins the Olympic gold medal in Seoul, South Korea.
1992	Henry Maske becomes world champion as a professional boxer in the light heavyweight division.

PURPOSE
OF FITNESS BOXING

Fitness boxing is an all-around series of exercises in which certain parts of training done by boxers (jumping rope, strength-training, punching, work on heavy and speed bags, and partner-training with padded mitts) are combined with elements of other types of sports (like aerobic exercises and stretching). This develops and improves strength, stamina, speed, agility, and coordination. Strength is necessary for working on the heavy bag; stamina is needed to sustain prolonged physical activity. Rope-jumping and punching drills increase speed, agility and coordination. The speed bag has to be hit quickly and accurately, and speed and accuracy are also important when hitting the gloves of your training partner. Both exercises are also excellent training for improving agility and concentration.

The fitness boxing exercises described in this book were designed to provide a holistic training program. While these exercises offer many different variations of a boxing-specific training, they are geared more to those who want to become fit. In selecting the exercises, we were guided more by fitness-related aspects than would be the case if this book was meant for training exclusively oriented to improve the performance of boxers.

BENEFITS OF FITNESS BOXING

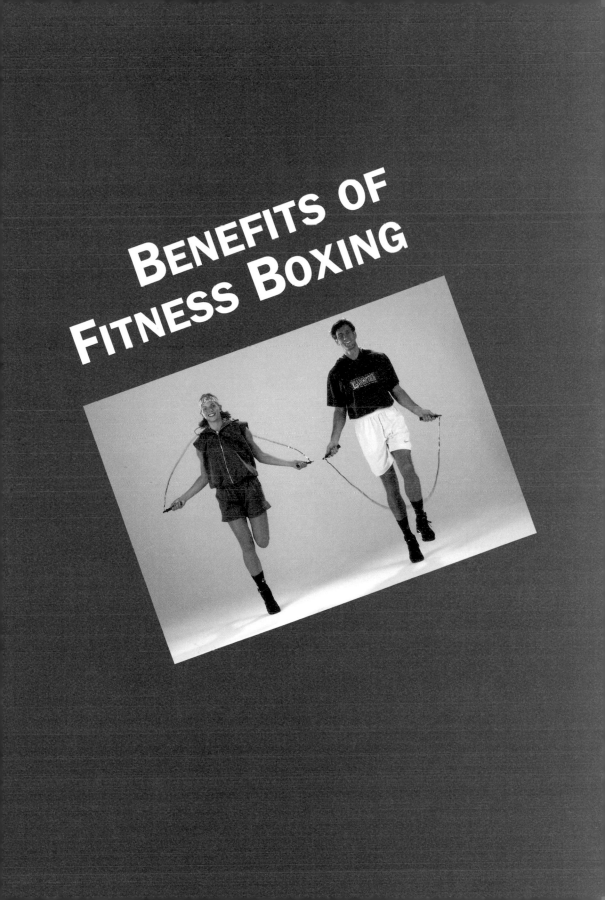

IMPROVED FITNESS THROUGH TRAINING

Anybody who is exercising for fitness usually has very definite expectations of what a training program should accomplish. In order to become more fit and well-conditioned, you must exercise to increase your stamina and strength, stretching ability, reaction time, and coordination. This will not only increase your performance level by, among other things, improving your ability to deal with fatigue, it also will make your body more attractive and improve your self-confidence.

Fitness boxing is particularly well-suited to improving motor skills.

To be physically fit means to have sufficient stamina, strength, and mobility to move smoothly, quickly, and correctly. Sports science states that a good athlete must possess a sufficient degree of the following elements of conditioning: stamina, strength, agility, speed and coordination. They represent the five essential building blocks of modern fitness training. (See Stemper/Wastl 1994, 6.)

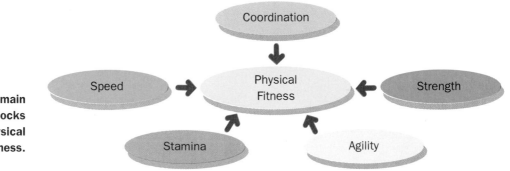

The main building blocks of physical fitness.

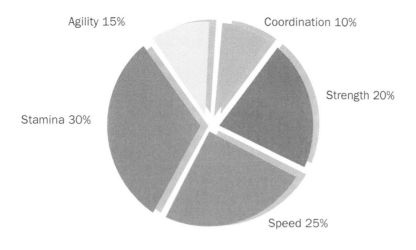

Agility 15%   Coordination 10%

Strength 20%

Stamina 30%

Speed 25%

The most important motor skills that provide the building blocks for boxing (from Jonath/Krempel 1991, 381)

The chart above shows how great a part each of the building blocks plays in producing a well-conditioned boxer. Note that stamina is the dominant building block. This means that overall stamina, in addition to good mobility and coordination, is necessary to carry out the constant evasive movements as a protection from the opponent's attack. Also of enormous importance is good "localized" strength in a boxer's arms and legs that enables him to consistently and successfully carry out his offenses in the first place. For a boxer's punches to have the required effect, there must be sufficient power behind them.

The effects boxing exercises have on the very basic motor skills is also important to those athletes who want to remain fit. Fitness boxing, in contrast to many other sports, is one of the few training regimens that does not concentrate on one particular motor skill, but improves a whole variety of skills. As described in more detail in the following chapters, it consists of powerful exercises with many repetitions and at different speeds. These exercises are complemented with other exercises that increase mobility and reaction time. All of these exercises are essential to achieve a good level of fitness.

An additional advantage of fitness boxing is that it contributes to a person's emotional well-being. It does this by strengthening his self-discipline and ability to concentrate not only through the training, but also through competition with an opponent. It improves your ability to react to the challenges in your environment.

REQUIREMENTS AND TRAINING EFFECTS

Psychological Effects

It has been shown that fitness boxing requires a person to be able to anticipate, react, and concentrate. These abilities are shaped particularly when he is training with a partner. This is because one must always be alert and react with lightning speed to deflect an opponent's punch and simultaneously recognize and take advantage of his defensive mistakes. All these movements, while very complex and demanding, must be focused and done with great precision. A proper stance and correct body and arm movements require good body coordination.

And in spite of the power and aggressiveness that is necessary for throwing a punch, one must be disciplined to avoid injuries. Of highest priority is the safety not only of yourself but also that of the partner. In addition, this type of aggressiveness requires great concentration because if you do not pay attention to your opponent's actions you will get hit and maybe even injured.

Conditioning Effects of Training

We have already mentioned that boxing exercises train all the basic motor skills. This can be said only about very few athletic activities. The real question is how fitness boxing compares to specific sport activities in terms of training effects. First of all, the type of athletic activity is of primary importance when gauging the effects of a training program because some increase stamina, other primarily increase strength, and yet others increase mobility. The table on the next page is a summary of well-known sports activities for amateurs. We have tried to indicate the training effects as they address individual motor skills. This includes information on which activity is suitable for particular age groups (with tips for people over 50) and to what degree their joints will be stressed.

Type of Sport	Training Effects					Suitability	
	Stamina	Strength	Speed	Agility	Coordi-nation	Stress to the joints	50 years old and up
Running	●●●	●	●	○	●	▲▲	○
Bicycling	●●●	●●	○	○	●	▲	●●○
Swimming	●●○	●○	○	●	●●	△	●●●
Bodybuilding	○	●●●	○	●●	●	▲△	○
Football	●●○	●	●●●	●	●●	▲▲▲	○
Basketball	●	●●	●●●	●●	●●●	▲▲△	○
Volleyball	○	●●	●●●	●●	●●●	▲▲	●
Tennis	○	●●	●●●	●	●●●	▲▲	●
Squash/ Badminton	●	●●	●●●	●●	●●●	▲▲▲	○
Circuit-training	●●●	●●●	●	●●	●●	▲	●●○
Fitness-boxing	●●○	●●	●●●	●●○	●●●	▲▲	○

●●● very good		●● good		● average		△/○ with moderation	
▲▲▲ very high		▲▲ high		▲ modest			

The table above shows, that relative to other athletic activities, fitness boxing plays a special role because almost no other athletic activity provides as many positive effects as fitness-oriented boxing exercises. This fact can be verified by the drawing on the next page, which compares several different types of sport activities and how they improve strength and mobility in the total body. It shows that fitness-boxing exercises, when compared to other types of sports, build strength and mobility to a very high degree. The upper and lower body are being developed equally. This is because weak muscles lead to poor legwork, which hinders mobility and puts limited power behind every punch. Consequently, all large muscles must be trained equally (including the muscles of the "weaker" side of the body).

Training effect and suitability of different types of sport for fitness athletes (according to Stemper/Wastl 1994, 8).

17

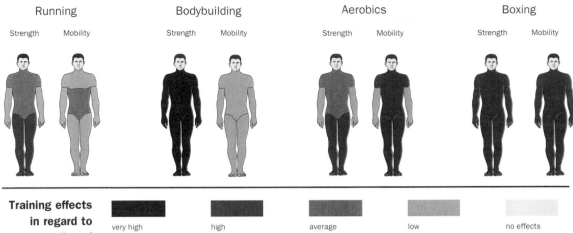

Running		Bodybuilding		Aerobics		Boxing	
Strength	Mobility	Strength	Mobility	Strength	Mobility	Strength	Mobility

very high	high	average	low	no effects

Training effects in regard to strength and mobility of the total musculature of the body, comparing boxing to running, bodybuilding, and aerobics (according to Gavin, 1989).

The drawing below shows how all major muscle groups are engaged when a straight punch is thrown with your hand. In the process, the entire body is used, not just the muscles in the upper and lower arm. A boxer puts his whole body mass behind a punch, whereby a significant portion of the power is transferred to the opponent or the heavy bag. If the punch misses its goal, the boxer, due to the weight of his own body, falls forward (see also Tittel 1994, 209).

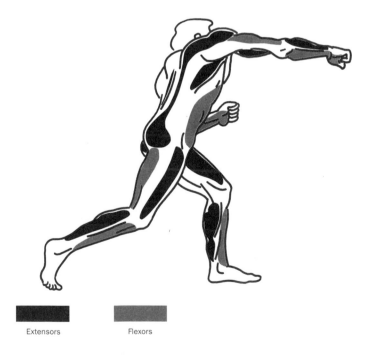

Muscle action during boxing (according to Tittel 1994, 210-211).

Extensors	Flexors

Boxing-specific action	Muscles Used
Leg movement • Forward, lateral or back muscles	Muscles for flexing toes, and thigh and buttock muscles
Avoidance movement of the body • weaving and rolling • ducking and diving	Large flexor muscles of the back, trunk muscles, straight stomach muscles, lateral stomach muscles and thigh muscles
Avoidance movement of the arm and shoulder • Shoulder and elbow blocking	Upper arm muscles, shoulder muscles, chest muscles
Type of hitting • Upward, head, and body hooks • Combination punching • Straight punch, cross-punch	Finger muscles, lower arm muscles, upper arm muscles, shoulder and chest muscles

Movement and muscles used during boxing (according to Jonath/Krempel 1991, 381).

The table above shows what kind of muscles or muscle groups are used during boxing-specific movements. But success is not limited to muscle development. Body shape is also improved. Since the training includes exercises that improve strength as well as stamina, visually recognizable body-shaping effects also became apparent over time. While stamina-increasing exercises primarily reduce body fat, strength-increasing exercises also add muscle mass. Basically, we can state that positive effects are the result when you engage in boxing-specific exercises without sparring (which is the case in fitness boxing).

The table on page 20 summarizes the physical demands placed on a boxer. Athletes who want to become totally fit will benefit greatly by adhering to fitness boxing exercises because they can improve somewhat in each of these areas. This is an effective training program, which has the long-range goal of maintaining good health.

Elements	General Demands	Boxing-Specific Characteristics
Conditioning	*Stamina:* • General aerobic endurance (improving and optimizing your cardiovascular system and strength)	• Prolonged rope-jumping or punching training
	Strength: • Maximum energy • Speed • Strength and stamina *Speed:* • Action/reaction speed	• Vigorous punches on heavy or speed bags, or with partner • Extended rope-jumping or punching exercises • Quick and precise *hits* on speed bag or with focus mitts
	Nimbleness: • Agility • Flexibility	• Consistent moves to avoid being hit by the opponent or moving back and forth
Coordination	• Combination skill	• Proper coordination of individual punching movements
	• Orientation skill	• Active confrontation with your partner (constantly changing distance and position)
	• Ability to judge movements	• Precise and finely tuned execution of part and whole movements on the basis of well-measured energy appropriate to the situation
	• Ability to react	• Timely and lightning-quick reaction to the action of the partner
	• Ability to balance	• Maintaining or reestablishing a secure stance and balance when under attack or after a quick movement
Cognitive Ability	• Discipline, staying power	• Self-discipline and discipline with partner
	• Preparing to endure • Concentration • Willpower • Self-control	• Self-control and concentration • Work/training • Appropriate reaction to the demands of the environment

Boxing's Physical Demands

The Basics of Boxing

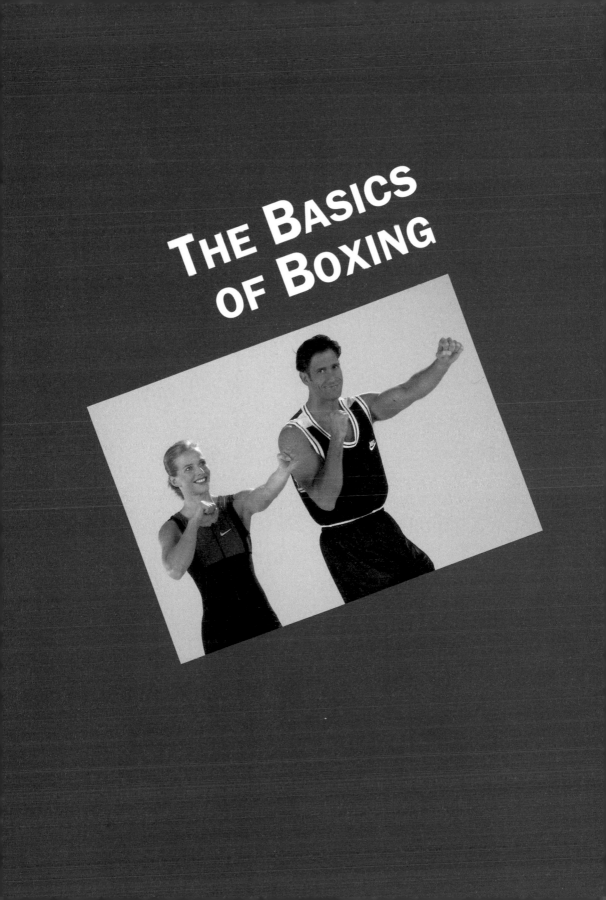

EQUIPMENT AND AIDS

As in any other sport, fitness boxing also requires appropriate basic equipment. We are not, however, talking about what a competitive boxer or members of a boxing club need because we are concentrating exclusively on boxing exercises for a fitness athlete, and the cost for the items needed for fitness athletes can be kept to a minimum.

Fitness-boxing workouts require neither a boxing ring nor a gymnasium. The space needed can be relatively small, and usually can be found in your own house. Clothing should be adapted to the prevailing temperature, be breathable, and allow for freedom of movement.

Since boxing requires a great deal of legwork, athletic shoes that fit well, absorb shock, and are slip-resistant play an important role because you will do a lot of jumping (such as when jumping rope). We recommend ankle-high aerobic, cross-training, or basketball shoes. Boxing boots are only good for competitive fights in the ring. They are not good for fitness exercises because they have very little cushion and protection.

Equipment Needed and Cost

Fitness boxing does not involve climbing into the ring, and thereby keeps the cost manageable. As far as clothing is concerned, walking or jogging shorts and a tee-shirt are really all that are needed. What follows is a summary of equipment with approximate costs:

Athletic shoes	$60-120
Jump rope	$4-40
Flexible rope	$18-30
Hand weights	$30 -70
Exercise mat	$12-30
Boxing bandages	$7-12
Boxing gloves	$30-120
Gloves	$12-90
Combination focus mitts	$60-92
Exercise focus mitts	$60-92
Heavy bag	$30-220
Speed bag	$30-120
Pulse-frequency measuring device	$100-120

If sparring exercises are part of the training program add, for safety reasons, protective head gear, a mouth guard, and an athletic protector. Boxing shoes are only necessary for competitions held in places that have wooden floors. Following is a list describing the cost of this equipment:

Boxing boots	$45–175
Head protector	$45–120
Athletic protector	$12–20
Mouth guard	$12

Heavy Bag

The best known and most important piece of equipment needed for boxing exercises is the heavy bag. It is a substitute for an opponent. The heavy bag is used to learn and practice combinations and different punching techniques. It is also used for other aspects of training, like learning to throw a series of punches, distance punching, and infight-interval punching, as well as improving your punching power.

The outer skin of the heavy bag is made of leather, linen, nylon, or very strong plastic. The bag should be about 32 inches long. In general, the heavy bag is stuffed tightly with old rags or cloth remnants. As an alternative, it is also possible to insert a smaller bag filled with sand inside the heavy bag where the space between the smaller bag and the outer skin is filled with horsehair or felt. Specialty shops carry bags that are already filled or empty heavy bags that you can stuff yourself.

Due to the weight and the powerful force with which the bags are hit during training, the heavy bag must be secured to the ceiling by a very strong and safe mechanism. The heavy bag should be suspended from the ceiling in such a way that it does not extend beyond your torso. The height of the heavy bag can be adjusted with a suspension chain.

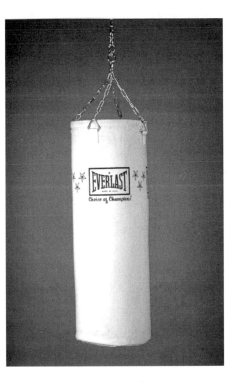

Speed Bag

The speed bag consists of a pear-shaped leather bag with a linen bag inside it that is filled with corn. This bag is considerably lighter than the heavy bag and extends from the ceiling at head height.

The speed bag is used for practicing quick punches and movements as well as different types of hits (straight hits, uppercuts, and combinations). It is also excellent for learning avoidance movements and for developing a sense for distance. Because this bag constantly moves back and forth at varying distances, it is also an excellent means of learning to coordinate punches and to improve legwork.

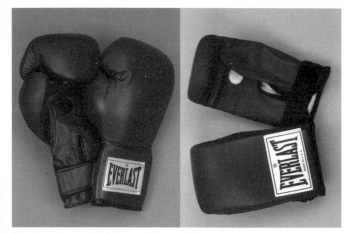

Boxing gloves (left) and gloves (right).

Boxing Gloves

Boxing gloves serve to protect the hands, to increase the area of impact, and to dampen the impact of the boxer's hands, which also protects the opponent. They are padded with horsehair, foam, or air. Boxing gloves come in different weight categories. Eight- and ten-ounce gloves are competition gloves. Heavier gloves may be used for training. Keep in mind that heavier gloves afford better protection and greater cushioning effect, but that punches are thrown more slowly.

Focus Mitts (Hand Cushions)

Focus mitts are gloves that have oval leather cushions inserted on their palm sides. They are the target for punching practice (see the photo on page 43). They are used when training with a partner, which is the closest you will come to an actual fight situation.

When using focus mitts, you can practice throwing punches and jabs at a moving target. This is an excellent way to practice precision, coordination, and combination punches. The trainer or partner, by continually moving his raised hand, challenges the student to constantly adjust his offense and counterpunches. If done with intensity this part of the training program comes very close to real competition.

When working with focus mitts, the trainer or partner, who represents the opponent, is better able to observe and correct the student. The photo below shows so-called combination focus mitts. These mitts are a compromise between normal focus mitts and boxing gloves. With these gloves, a partner or trainer is able to counterpunch and quickly point out possible errors in defense. Partners can alternate between punching and counterpunching, constantly moving about, which produces as close to a real boxing match as possible.

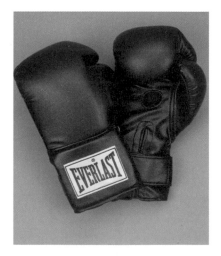

Ball Gloves

Ball gloves are leather gloves that are thinner and lighter than boxing gloves and are used exclusively for practice on boxing equipment. They are supposed to protect the skin from abrasions and other injuries (see photo on the bottom of page 24).

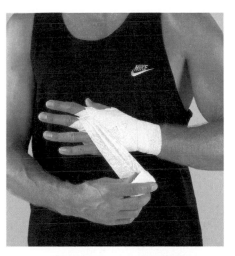

Boxing Bandages

Boxing bandages are special elastic wraps worn under the gloves. They give good support for the fist, and reduce the danger of injuries to the hands, fingers and thumbs. Hands are bandaged in different ways. It is important that the wrists, the bones of the middle hands, and the knuckles are well-supported. In the photos that are shown on the right, the wrist is bandaged first. The bandage is wrapped around each finger once and back to the wrist again. Finally, the bandage should be wrapped several times around the knuckles and the hand.

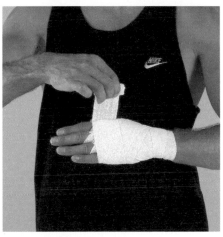

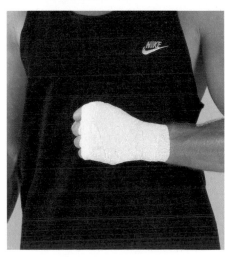

Flexible Rope

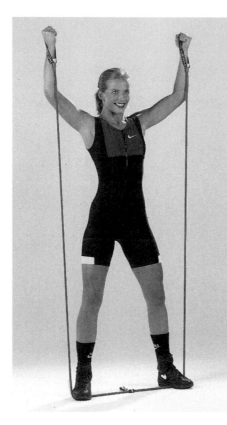

Elastic rope comes in different sizes and has a handle at each end. It is used to increase strength and stamina, and can be used during punching exercises.

Jump Rope

A jump rope is absolutely essential for boxing training. A jump rope is made from rubber, hemp, or steel and has a grip on each end. The length is adjustable. How the rope and the handles are joined together is important. This connection must allow the rope to move easily and should not slow it down. The heavier the rope, the faster the rotation. Rope-jumping, also called rope skipping, is a very demanding part of a boxing workout. It improves endurance, coordination, and agility, and builds strong leg muscles.

Heavy Hands

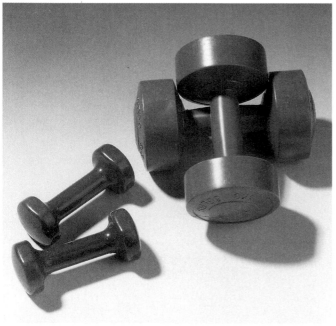

Heavy Hands are small handheld weights that are a sensible addition to every strength/endurance training. They are used during all phases of shadow-boxing and circuit-training.

BOXING BASICS

Boxing Stance

The goal in boxing is to throw as many punches at your opponent while sustaining as few as possible to yourself. The target is the front of the upper body (above the waistline, excluding the arms) and the head. This means that the boxer has to assume a stance that allows him to hit his opponent from any position while avoiding being hit and blocking the opponent's punches.

The basic boxing stance, the set stance, is the characteristic posture a boxer assumes before and after every action. In this stance, he is always ready for action. The stance allows him to take lightning-fast offensive and defensive actions. This posture should be loose and relaxed, to avoid becoming prematurely tired.

Depending on which is the punching hand, several different stances are possible. The punching hand is the hand that delivers the more powerful punches. The leading hand prepares for offensive action and defends the boxer. If the right hand is the punching hand, the boxer will usually punch from a left stance, in which the left hand and the left foot are in a forward position. The left hand is then the leading hand. For left-handed people, it is the reverse.

The following discussion describes the left stance because most people are right - handed.

The leg position for the right-

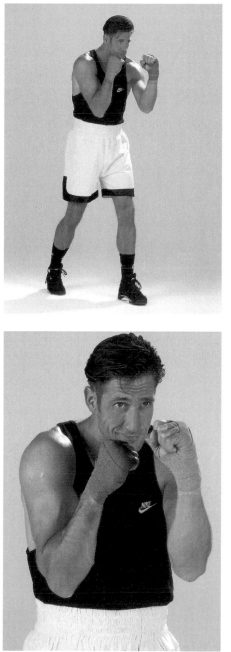

handed boxer is as follows: stand with your feet shoulder-width apart, your right foot slightly in front of your left foot, toes pointing straight ahead. Your left heel should be slightly above the ground, and your right foot flat on the ground. Your body weight should be distributed evenly; rest on the ball of your feet. Your knees should be slightly bent. Your upper body should be leaning forward slightly and, corresponding to the placement of the feet, your left shoulder should point slightly forward. Your elbows should point down, and should be held close to your body. Your punching fist should be in front of your chin, and your leading hand should be held head-high in a position that corresponds to the foot set forward. The back of your hands and underarm should

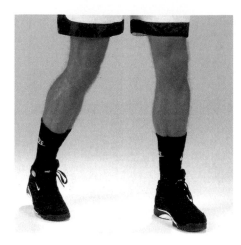

Leg position in left stance.

create a straight line and point to the outside. Your first should be closed, and your thumb placed at the second joint of your middle finger. Having a solid stance and moving easily in all directions are prerequisites for developing offensive and definesive moves.

Legwork

First-rate legwork is important for boxing successfully because a boxer must constantly change his positions and be ready to carry out offensive and defensive actions. Not only should a boxer's stance allow him to move smoothly and quickly, it must also be steady and solid so he can throw punches effectively and not lose his balance when blocking an opponent's attacks.

The drawing of the footprints on the following page shows the basic sequence of steps of a boxer: the

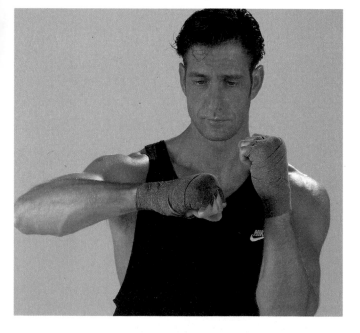

The back of the hand and the underarm are creating a straight line.

foot in the forward position is placed on the ground first. While in the boxing posture, move your foot flat on to the floor forward about an inch. Then move your other foot forward also until both feet are back in their original positions.

Throughout the movement, your feet should move flat against the floor so that you can quickly assume a solid stance and be able to throw punches effectively from every position. The steps are short and subtle and almost impossible to recognize by the opponent. Remember, your first contact with the floor always is with the balls of your feet. From this "fighting stance," it is also possible to jump in all directions, always close to the floor and on the balls of your feet. In a way, the boxer is "dancing" around his opponent.

An effective boxing stance occurs when leg and arm movements are combined. Stepping and hitting take place at the same time: the fist is hitting the target as the foot is making contact with the floor.

Tip: A large mirror is very helpful during practice, not only to learn to control movements, but also to learn the basic body stance and the legwork involved.

Punching

In boxing, it is particularly important that punches are thrown quickly and from a relaxed posture. When you throw a punch, it is not only the muscles of your arm, but your whole body that is contracted. As soon as you throw a punch, with the fastest possible speed pull your punching arm back quickly to assume a defensive posture.

The diagram on the following page is a summary of different boxing punches.

Boxing Punches

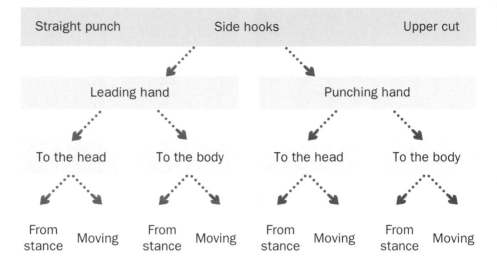

Straight punch	Side hooks	Upper cut

Leading hand	Punching hand

To the head	To the body	To the head	To the body

From stance	Moving	From stance	Moving	From stance	Moving	From stance	Moving

"Distances"

"Distance" is the range of the punch in relation to the opponent. Depending on the type of punch, the technique, and a boxer's physical condition, boxers fight at different ranges. We distinguish between wide range, half range, and close range (almost body on body).

Straight Punch with the Leading Hand

A straight punch with the leading hand has many diverse tactical uses. It often is a preparation for offensive action. It establishes the proper distance, continuously keeps the opponent occupied, constricts the range of the opponent's action, and often stops his offense. We discuss here only the punch from a left stance. From the set stance the left arm is thrown quickly and

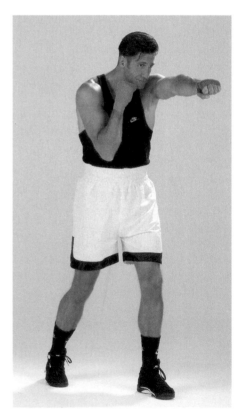

forcefully forward. Body weight is shifted to the front foot, and a simultaneous shift forward of the shoulder and hip on the same side supports the hit. The distance should be such that the outstretched arm just about reaches its target. The fist moves in a straight line to the target and straight back again as a safeguard.

The back of the hand and the lower arm are in a straight line and turned up at the moment of impact. The left shoulder moves towards the chin for protection. The right fist serves as a safeguard in front of the chin, and the elbow is close to the body. The right foot rests on the ball of the foot and supports the punch. Immediately after the punch, the fist is pulled back to its original position.

The straight hook is carried out with the leading hand as quickly as possible, but with varying degrees of power: either as a hard left shot or a quick jab. A jab is a light but very quickly thrown straight punch of the leading hand. Overall, the jab is very effective and can combine defensive and offensive actions and, in addition, can score points and be very distracting to the opponent.

The straight leading hand can also be used for body punches. The movements are the same as the sequence discussed above except the upper body is bent forward more and, during the punch, is moving slightly to the right.

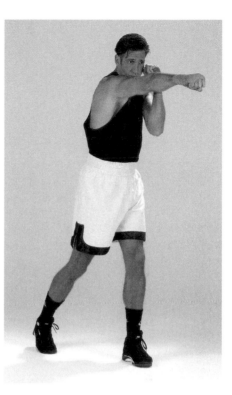

Straight Punch with the Punching Hand

This technique is designed to put pressure on the opponent with the punching hand. Without reaching back, the arm moves straight forward from the chin. The head and the shoulder on the same side twist forward to support the action.

The back leg is stretched, with the ball of the foot pushing into the floor. This shifts the body weight to the front foot, with the result that the whole weight of the body is put behind the punch. Because of the force with which the ball of the foot is pushed into the floor, energy moves from the foot through the leg and the body to the fist. As is the case when throwing a straight punch with the leading hand, the arm is stretched out with the back of the hand straight and pointing up. After impact, the punching arm is immediately pulled back for protection. During the punch, the shoulder and the punching hand guard the chin, and the leading hand guards the head and the upper body. When a straight hook is thrown to the body, the knees are bent more.

Side Hooks with the Punching Hand

Hooks are very effective punches to the head and the body from a medium distance. They are bent-arm blows delivered from the side. While the boxer must move closer to his opponent and pay more attention to his own defense, side hooks to the head allow him to circumvent his opponent's defenses.

What follows is a description of the side hook from a left stance. From a secure defensive stance, the hitting arm is opened up approximately 90° degrees but with the elbow still close to the body. The right shoulder now turns with lightning speed forward, and the elbow moves up to shoulder height. The fist moves in a circular motion to the head of the opponent, with the elbow bent.

At the moment of impact the back of the fist is pointing slightly up, and in a straight line with the lower arm. The right shoulder is rotated when the ball of the foot is forcefully pushed against the floor and the right hip is stretched. Body weight is shifted to the leading leg, and the body is tightened. The leading hand

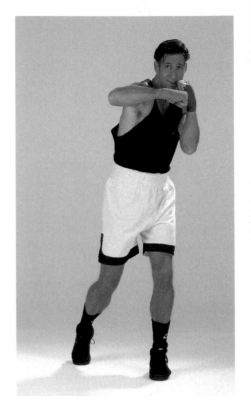

protects the head and upper body during the punch.

When you are throwing a series of punches, your upper body should be shifting slightly to the left, to avoid being hit by your opponent with his leading hand. When you are throwing a side hook to the body, your upper body should be bent forward more, and your legs bent more from the hips and knee joints. Since this weakens the defense somewhat, you must pull back your hitting arm and straighten your body quickly.

Make sure that your punches are explosive, your hips are engaged, and your body weight is shifted. To avoid injury, it is essential that your hands and wrists are held in a fixed position.

Side Hooks with the Leading Hand

Without reaching back, thrust the fist of your leading hand forward in the direction of your opponent's head while quickly rotating your upper body, pressing your front leg down, and rotating your hip on the same side. As a result, shift your body weight to your rear foot. The sequence of arm movements is similar to those used for the side hook with your punching hand. To better bridge the distance and put more power into the punch, you can push off your front foot and take a quick step.

For a side hook to the body, increase the rotation of your upper body and lean more to the right side.

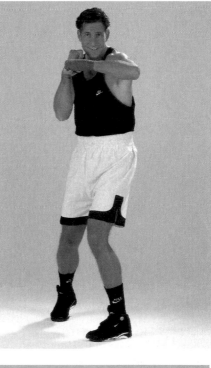

Uppercut

The uppercut is carried out at close range. The boxer punches and immediately pulls back his arm for defense in one continuous movement.

From a head-on boxing stance, drop the lower part of your punching arm until the upper and lower parts of your arm are at a right angle. Your fist and the back of your hand should point down. From this position, thrust your arm forward and in the direction of your opponent's head. Body hooks are thrown more straight ahead.

Since the uppercut is thrown with your arm closer to your body, the power of the punch is created by engaging your whole body.

When making an uppercut with your punching hand, your body weight during the initial movement

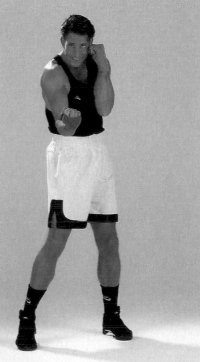

should be over the rear leg. Straighten this leg, rotate your hip and shoulder on the same side forward, and turn the heel of your rear leg to the outside while your arm is thrusting forward. Shift your body weight to the leg in front (see the photo on the bottom of page 33). Since, in the course of these punches, the boxer's body remains unprotected, the arm that is not involved in the punching must take over the defense and be held in front of the chin. The danger of being hit by your opponent is considerable, which is why the uppercut is seldom used as an individual punch but usually only as part of a combination of punches.

Defense

The basic rule in boxing is to throw punches without getting hit. Therefore, in addition to the hitting techniques described, we will

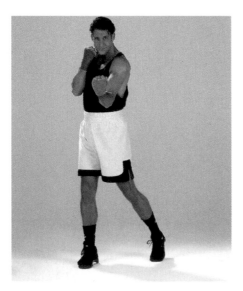

discuss several different forms of defensive actions that are available. In boxing, there is a difference between *active defense*, i.e., counterpunching or counteroffense, and *passive* defense, which has nothing to do directly with punching or counteroffense.

Blocking

Blocking is a technique that deflects an opponent's punch to those parts of the body that are not considered targets (hands, lower arm, elbows, upper arm, and shoulder). We distinguish between several different types of blocking. They are as follow:
1. Guarding your head. Protecting your head with your fist kept on the right or left side of your head.
2. Elbow block. Protecting your body with your lower arm and elbow by slightly rotating your body in the direction of the punch.
3. Double-blocking. Holding your fists in front of your slightly bent head and pulling your elbows in front of your body. This in effect protects every potential target.
4. Shoulder block. Protecting your chin from the side with your shoulder, which is pulled up.

Parry

Parry is a technique that absorbs, deflects, or beats back an opponent's punch. A punch can be deflected to the inside, outside, or upward. A punch can also be blocked by checking the direction of the movement. When the boxer is successfully beating back an opponent's punch, it is called counterpunching.

Blocking	Parry	Avoidance Movements	Evasive Movements
head block	to the inside	ducking	stepping
elbow block	to the outside	riding it out	sideways
double block	diving	swinging	stepping back
shoulder block		rolling upward	jumping back

Avoidance Movements

Avoidance movements are all movements that are primarily carried out by moving the upper body. They include:

1. *Ducking.* Bending forward left/right to get out of the way of a punch.

2. *Swinging.* Bending to the side and away from the punch.

3. *Riding it out.* Bending back and away from the punch. Your body weight should be shifted back. This is a good position for counterpunching because your muscles are tightened and your opponent's still in the contact zone.

4. *Diving.* Lowering your body by bending your knees to escape the punches.

5. *Rolling.* This consists of bending your upper body to either side depending on the direction of your opponent's hooks, knees slightly bent, and "diving" under the punch so that you can counterpunch on the opposite side of your opponent by straightening your legs. This is a good defensive technique against uppercuts targeted to the side of your head.

Evasive Movements

Evasive movements are used to avoid an opponent's actions through active legwork (steps and jumps), to get out of reach of the opponent, and to create a favorable offensive position. A variation of these movements are evasive side-step movements that consist of stepping and jumping back.

It is important when making evasive movements to always maintain a favorable offensive position because moving too far away puts you so far from your opponent that direct counter-punching becomes impossible.

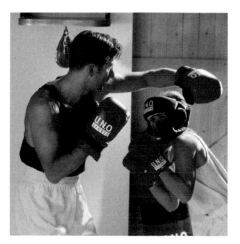

Shadowboxing

Shadowboxing is a type of training in which all punches, or punching combinations, and movements you have learned are used against an imaginary opponent. Smooth and fluid legwork, good blocking, and clean punches are important. To better control and observe your workout, practice in front of a large mirror. Mirrors are used not only by beginners but also by more-advanced athletes because you get immediate feedback on whether the movement is being done properly.

The objective of these imaginary fights is to combine punches and defensive techniques, in order to create offensive combinations from a protected position. In addition, it is a means of practicing specific tactics. Shadowboxing is also a very effective conditioning training because every movement is carried out quickly, under control, and with great concentration.

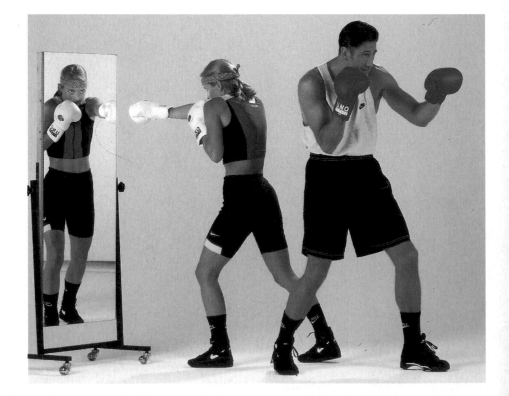

PROPER TRAINING PROGRAMS

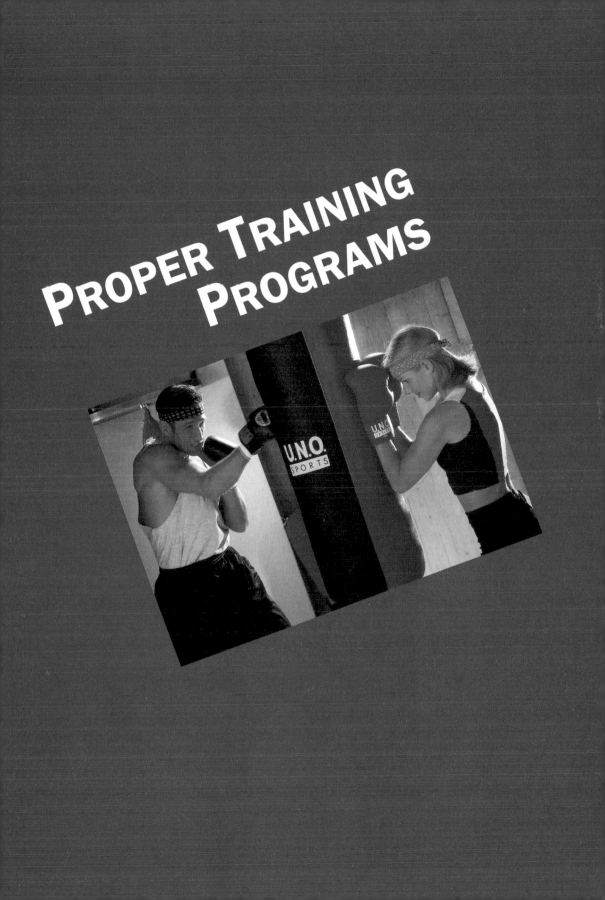

CHOICE OF EXERCISES

The previously listed training effects will be accomplished only when the exercises chosen are done properly and sensibly. The stress load should neither be too high nor too low, and should always be in proper relation to rest periods.

Those who want to start fitness boxing should first choose simple exercises and incorporate boxing-specific exercises over time. Exercises for the beginner should not be too demanding in terms of technique, skill, and coordination.

In addition, make sure when choosing your exercise routine that anatomical features such as your tendons, ligaments, joints, and spine are not exercised in the wrong way and that the risk of injuries inflicted by your partner are minimized. Otherwise, the whole workout will prove counterproductive, and result in diminished fitness through injuries rather than improved fitness.

For that reason, we have made sure when we established the training programs that the exercises are physiologically correct and that boxing-specific punching is only done on the heavy bag and the speed bag. Training with a partner is, therefore, done with focus mittens rather than through sparring. We wanted to be certain that training will bring the intended results with the smallest possible risks.

Conditioning Training

Boxing training also should include all the basic exercises needed to improve conditioning, that is, strength, stamina, speed, and mobility. Training to improve mobility can be accomplished best when it incorporates exercises we have presented on pages 43 to 78. These exercises include specific stretching exercises as part of the warm-up and cooldown programs.

For strengthening exercises, we recommend a circuit-training program like the one used in our boxing-circuit program. Jumping rope is particularly effective for improving stamina and strength. Punching exercises with your partner are particularly effective for improving speed and jumping ability.

The training program we have chosen (on pages 84-90) takes these considerations into account.

Coordination Exercises

The exercise programs that we have chosen for boxing workouts also improve coordination. One very good means of improving general coordination is jumping rope. Punching exercises with a partner improve specific abilities like ducking and diving.

Exercising with heavy and speed bags forces a person to constantly move with precise and coordinated leg, body, and punching movements that have appropriate power for the situation at hand. When training with a partner, each person must be able to react at any moment with lightning speed to the actions of his partner, must constantly be on the move to avoid his opponent's attack, and must always stay on his feet. This will also improve a person's ability to react and to keep his equilibrium.

To increase your coordination, use the Boxing for Professionals program on page 86, and the more technically oriented Technique and Power program on page 89.

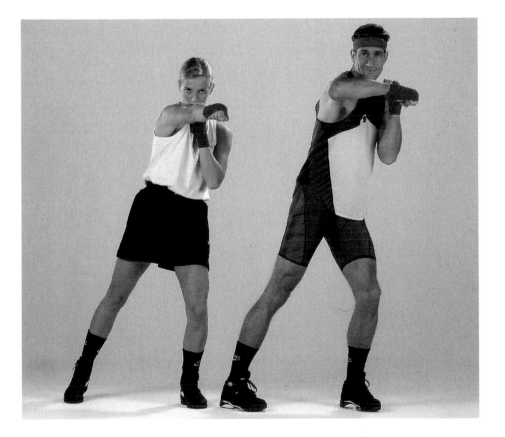

EXERCISE PROGRAM

Conditioning and Coordination Exercises

Determining an exact boxing exercise program is not easy. If you want to increase your stamina, you must do exercises at a slower tempo but with more repetitions. If you want to increase strength, increase the degree of difficulty and use additional weights. Also reduce the number of repetitions or shorten exercise periods. When training to increase speed, as when training for coordination, pay special attention to increase the speed and improve the precision of your movements.

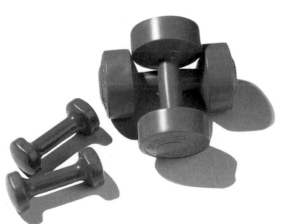

Interval Training

Since boxing workouts consist of several different programs, the exercise periods and the subsequent resting periods can be of different durations. The relationship between the exercises and rest periods may, however, also depend on your present condition and your goals.

Untrained athletes and beginners should in the beginning establish an exercise/ratio of 1:1 (20 seconds exercising and 20 seconds resting). Well-conditioned and advanced athletes can change to a 2:1 ratio (30 seconds of exercises and 15 seconds of rest, or 2 minutes of exercise and 1 minute of rest). Finally, a ratio of exercise and rest periods may, like in actual boxing competition, be increased to 3:1 (3 minutes of exercises and 1 minute of rest). This, however, as has already been mentioned, depends greatly on the exercise program you have chosen. For clarification, we have summarized the various exercise/rest ratios for different fitness-boxing exercises.

Fitness- Boxing Exercise	Speed of Movements		Exercise Period		Rest Period	
	Beginner	Advanced	Beginner	Advanced	Beginner	Advanced
Aerobic Boxing	swift	fast	20 sec.	30. sec	20. sec	15 sec
Jumping Rope	swift	swift	5–7min.	10 min.	none	none
Boxing Circuit	swift	swift/fast	20 sec.	30 sec.	20 sec.	15 sec.
Punching	swift/ fast	fast/ explosive	2 min.	3 min.	1 min.	1 min.
Partner-Training	slow/ swift	swift/ fast	2 min. (changing partner every 30 sec.)		30 sec.	
Stretching (Mobility Training)	slow/ holding	slow/ holding	20 sec. holding	20 sec. holding	10 sec.	10 sec.

Mobility Training

The stress load when exercising for improved mobility needs to be looked at separately because muscles can be stretched in many different ways. As a preparation for boxing-related workouts, we recommend active stretching exercises. These should always be done very gently, with slight pulling and bouncing movements. Jerky movements can lead to injuries and reduce the stretching effect. For the warm-up and cooldown exercises, we recommend passive stretching. Here, stretching is slow and careful, and each stretch is held for about 10 to 30 seconds. The muscle will slowly relax, and more stretching is possible.

Controlling Exercise Load

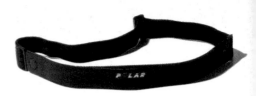

During boxing workouts, it is also important that the exercise load is neither too much nor too little. An appropriate exercise load for a beginner is one in which the activities are strenuous, but pleasant. Those with more experience can exercise until exhaustion if they stick to the required rest periods. You can also gauge your exercise load by observing your breathing. While your breathing markedly increases during training, your breathing rhythm should still be even.

The best way to measure the affects of the exercise program on your body is by checking your pulse. For a beginner, the pulse rate at the end of a fitness-boxing workout should not be higher than 170 beats per minute (minus his age). More advanced athletes can raise this to approximately 180 beats per minute (minus age). Depending on the type of training program, in boxing-specific training the pulse rate may also be slightly higher.

The easiest way to measure your pulse is by placing your index and middle fingers on your carotid artery or wrist. Immediately after the exercise, count your pulse for 10 seconds and multiply the result by 6. A precise reading of a pulse rate, however, is only possible with an electronic measuring device (see photo).

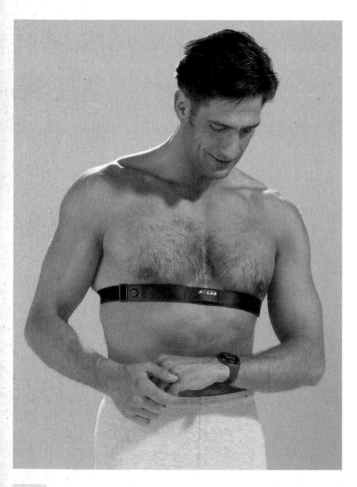

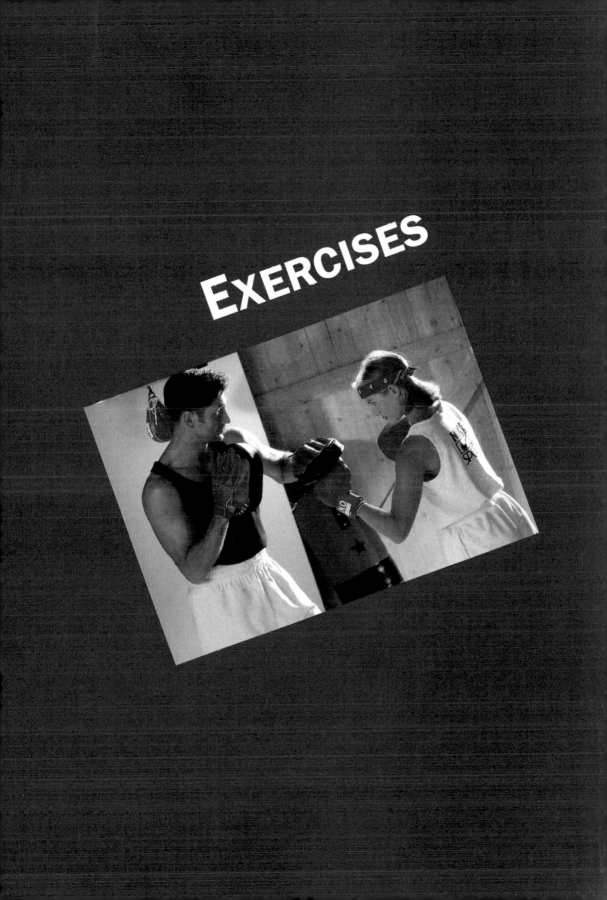

EXERCISES

WARM-UP

Warm-up exercises increase your body temperature and prepare you for the increased athletic activity to come. Slowly increasing the intensity of the exercise stimulates the circulatory system, breathing, and metabolism, and improves the transport of oxygen in your body. Warm-up exercises make the joints more flexible and stretch muscles, preparing the way for an effective workout. They also improve coordination and prepare a person mentally for the workout.

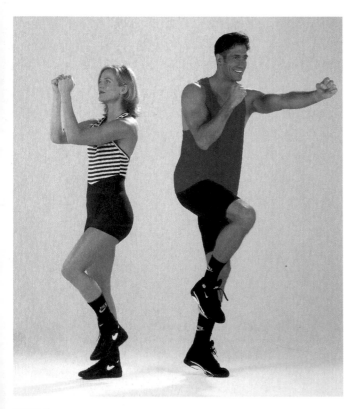

WARM-UP 1

Running in Place and Boxing: Begin by walking in place in a relaxed fashion with your arms in a boxing position. Alternately thrust your fists forward and back again quickly, and every now and then down to the leg in the forward position. Increase speed until you reach a gentle jog (see right figure in photo on this page). It is important to always keep your knees slightly bent and to set your feet on the floor gently.

Variations:
   1. Do the same exercises, but this time lift your knees higher and your fists up to your head and forward.
   2. Run in place, relaxed, moving your arms while they are bent together at right angles in front of your chest at shoulder level. Your fists should point up (see left figure in photo on this page).
   3. Run in place, relaxed, while circling your outstretched arms at shoulder level.
   4. Run in place, relaxed, while your arms, bent at right angles, move together or alternately up and forward.

WARM-UP 2

Bending Knees and Boxing: Keep your legs shoulder-width apart, your knees slightly bent (and toes pointing slightly to the outside), and your arms at right angles in front of your upper body for protection. Now, bend and alternately straighten each leg, alternately pushing your fists forward and quickly back again.

It is important that you do the knee bends slowly, and keep your body muscles contracted and back straight. During the bending phase, keep your knees above your feet and in the stretching position. Do not straighten your knees completely; this way, you can avoid unnecessary stress to knee and hip joints.

Variations:

1. Do the same exercise, but this time raise your outstretched arms to shoulder level. When stretching your legs, bring your arms up and touch your hands above your head. When bending your knees, return your arms to their original positions.

2. Do the same exercise, but this time punch your fists alternately straight upwards.

WARM-UP 3

Heel Lifts: Assume the set position with your feet hip-width apart. Hold your arms in front of your upper body for protection. Now, hop in place. While hopping, alternately bend the lower parts of your left and right legs back. That is, take a short hop with your right foot and your left leg bent at the knee, and land on both feet.

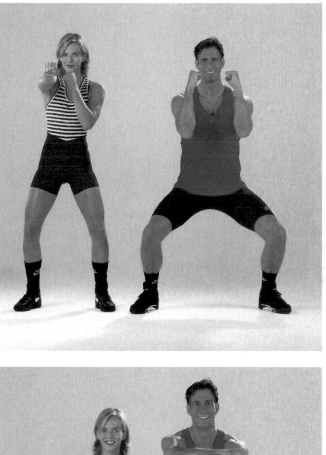

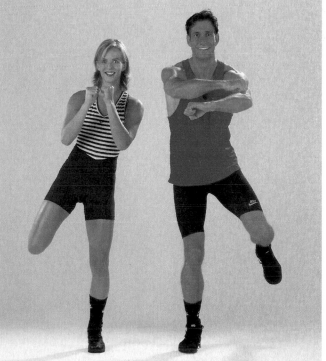

Then take a short hop with your left foot and your right leg bent at the knee, and land on both feet, etc. (see the left figure in the photo on the bottom of page 45).

Variations:

1. Do the same exercise, but this time move your arms, bent at right angles and at shoulder level, down in front of your body together, and then back again (fists pointing forward).

2. Do the same exercise, but this time cross your arms, bent at right angles and at shoulder level, in front of your chest and back again, fists pointing forward (see the right figure in the photo on the bottom of page 45).

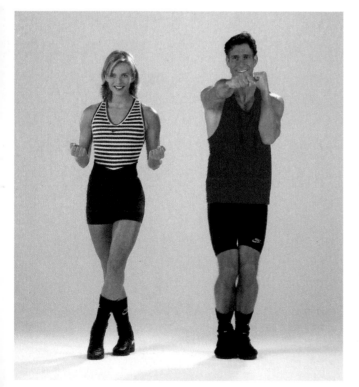

3. Do the same exercise, but this time move your arms together, bent at right angles and at shoulder level, in front of your chest and back to their original positions.

WARM-UP 4

Sidestep Boxing: With your feet hip-width apart, move your left or right leg to the side and place the other leg behind it. After another sidestep to the same side, place your other leg next to your lead leg. Allow your arms to swing in the same rhythm, keeping your fists tight. When sidestepping, bend your lower arm 90 degrees, contracting your biceps muscles, and move your straight arm downward (see the left figure in the photo on this page).

Variations:

1. Do the same exercise, but this time hold your bent arms as protection in front of your upper body and push your left and right arms alternately forward. After every fourth step, go into a crouch (see the right figure in the photo on this page).

2. Do the same exercise, but this time throw forward punches after every second step and later after every step.

WARM-UP 5

Stretching exercises: See the stretching exercise program on pages 76 to 78.

AEROBIC BOXING

Aerobic boxing is a special exercise that combines boxing and aerobic elements. It increases conditioning, coordination, mobility, and total body strength. If done to music with a quick beat, this exercise is particularly enjoyable. When engaging in aerobic boxing, it is important always to maintain good muscle tension.

AEROBIC BOXING 1

Step-Touch Boxing: Assume a set position with your feet hip-width apart and your knees slightly bent. Take one step to the side with either your right or left leg (a sidestep), and then pull your other leg towards it, just touching the floor. When your foot is on the ground, go into a slight crouch. Your arms should be in a defensive position. Every time a foot touches the ground, throw a straight punch towards the leg that supports the weight of your body.

It is important that your knees always remain slightly bent.

Variations:

1. Relax your arms and keep them close to your body. When your feet touch and your knees are bent, also bend your lower arms up and forward with their muscles contracted. The back of your hands should point down.

2. Throw a straight punch, and take a step forward with the leg on the same side.

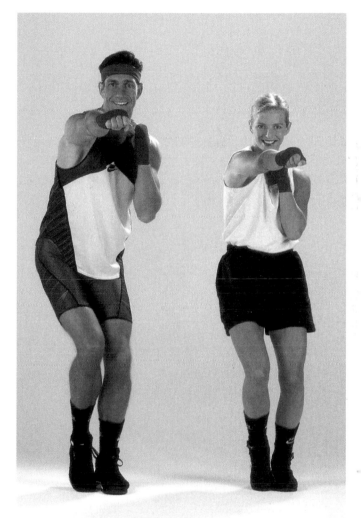

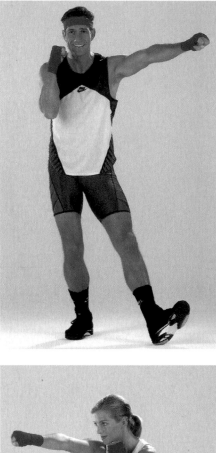

AEROBIC BOXING 2

Heel-Touch Boxing: Assume a set position with your feet hip-width apart. Now, alternately take a step and touch your heel either forward or to the side. Your body weight should always be over the supporting leg. Place your fists on your hips for support. *It is important that your back and stomach muscles remain contracted.*

Variations:

   1. With each touch, throw your fist on the same side forward (see top photo).

   2. With each touch, push both arms forward at the same time.

   3. With each side touch, push your arm on the same side either to the right or left.

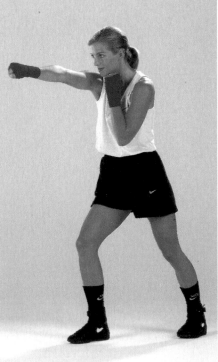

AEROBIC BOXING 3

Step-Jump Boxing: Assume a walking stance and raise your arms for protection. Jump with both legs at the same time and change the position of your legs in midair. Land on the floor on both feet. When landing, throw the same-side fist forward to the leg that is in front. You may bounce twice between each jump.

Variations:

   1. With your arms close to your body on each side, bend and stretch each arm with the arm muscles contracted.

   2. Lift your arms for protection, fists pointing inside. Now, lift your lower arms alternately.

AEROBIC BOXING 4

Squat Boxing: Assume a set position with your feet hip-width apart. Hold your arms in a boxing posture. Alternately lunge to the side with the weight of your body equally distributed over both bent legs. After each lunging step, return to your original position. At each side step, throw a straight punch forward.

AEROBIC BOXING 5

Knee Lifts with Arms: Assume a set position with your legs hip-width apart. Alternately pull one knee up high (knee lift). *It is important that the leg that supports the body weight always remain slightly bent.*

Variations:

1. Hold your arms straight over your head. With every knee lift, move your fists down and together at the back of your knee (see the left figure in the bottom photo).

2. Keep your bent arms at their sides at shoulder level, your elbows pointing out and fists forward. During each knee lift, cross your fists in front of your body (see the right figure in the bottom photo).

3. Bend your arms and hold them at shoulder level, elbows pointing out, fists pointing up. With each knee lift, alternately move your opposite elbow to your knee.

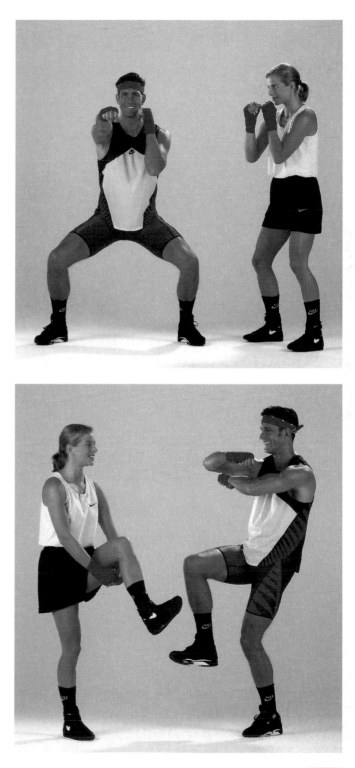

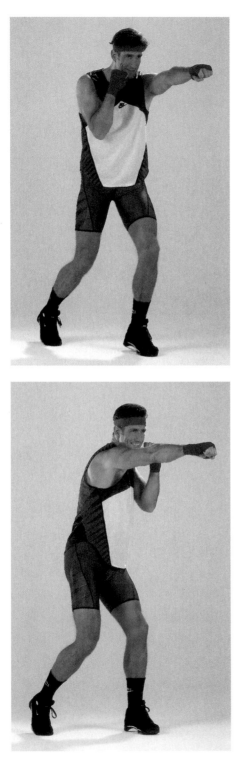

AEROBIC BOXING 6

Boxing Steps Forward/Backward:
Assume a set position, your arms in their defensive positions. With short steps (boxing steps), jump forward and backwards. Always touch the floor first with the foot that is in back. Throw light and quick jabs with your leading hand every time the foot in front touches the floor, and immediately pull your arm back for protection. *It is important to quickly reestablish contact with the floor.*

Variation:
   1. Take two quick boxing steps forward with every jab, and then two steps back.

AEROBIC BOXING 7

Falling Steps with Different Combinations: Assume a set position. Shift your body weight from your right to left leg. At that point, lift your right heel and then place your left foot flat on the ground. Your body weight now rests on your left leg. Lift your left heel and place your right foot fully on the ground. By lifting your heel and standing on the other foot, you seem to be falling somewhat to the side, which enables you to put your whole body weight behind your punch. When throwing the punch, rotate your shoulder and hip to the side while lifting your heel. Make a forward jab. *It is important to shift your body weight.*

Variations:
   1. Do the same exercise, but use a hook instead of a jab.
   2. Do the same exercise, but throw two jabs or hooks in succession (double punch).

AEROBIC BOXING 8

Side-Lunge Boxing: Assume a set position. Alternately step to the side with your right and left feet and back again. Throw jabs with the arm on the same side of the leg that does not support your body weight (see the left figure in the top photo). Move your hand back immediately after the jab, for protection. This exercise can be used with all punching techniques.

It is important that your knees be slightly bent and your body weight always be shifted to the supporting leg.

Variation:

1. Do the same exercise, but now use hooks instead of jabs (see the right figure in the top photo).

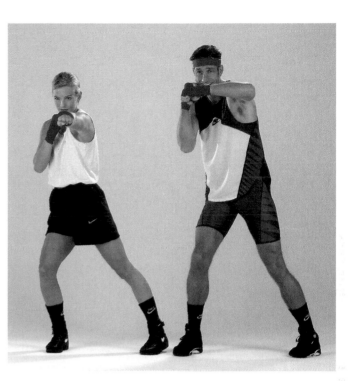

AEROBIC BOXING 9

Back-and-Forth Ducking: Assume a set position. Throw a jab while taking a short step forward with the leg that is in front. When stepping back, move your arms immediately back too, for protection. Now, step back with the leg that is in back and lift your right arm for protection by using your elbow to block an imaginary punch. Then return to your basic stance.

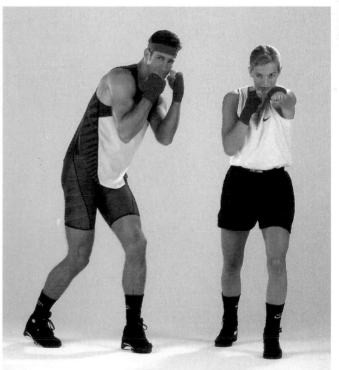

JUMPING ROPE

Jumping rope is an important part of fitness-oriented boxing workouts. It increases stamina, strengthens leg muscles, and improves coordination and mobility. It can be practiced anywhere, even in a small room. All you need is a jump rope. *It is important to wear ankle-high athletic shoes with a well-padded sole. Due to danger of injuries, never jump rope with bare feet. A flat, springy floor surface is ideal.*

To find the proper length of the rope, stand with your feet together on the rope and pull the handles up until your arms bend at a right angle. The length of the rope can be adjusted by either putting knots in

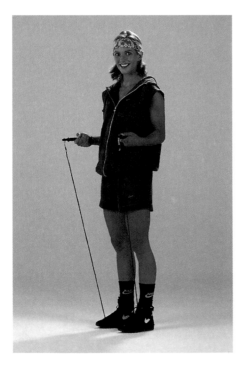

the appropriate places or using the mechanism that sometimes is built into the handles. Do a few practice jumps to make sure that the rope swings properly. In-between jumps are the same as basic jumps.

JUMPING ROPE 1

Basic Jumps: Assume the basic stance. Place the rope under your heels. Hold the ends of the rope at the handles. Swing the rope by moving your lower arms in circles and over your head. When the rope is touching the floor, jump over it with your feet close together.

Push off and land on the balls of your feet. Jump in a relaxed fashion and almost exclusively from your ankle joints. When landing, quickly roll your feet back to your heels. This ensures a soft landing, and the stress on the joints and spine is minimized. Jump only slightly off the ground, just enough for the rope to move underneath your feet.

Keep the upper part of your arms close to your body, and the lower parts of your arms pointed to the outside. The rope is kept in motion exclusively by wrist action. Keep your head straight, and do not lift your shoulders. *It is important to maintain a certain tension throughout your body.*

Variations:

1. Do the same exercise but with one extra jump while the rope is still in the air.

2. Assume your original stance and rest the rope in front of your feet. Now, swing the rope backwards over your head, and jump backwards over the rope.

JUMPING ROPE 2

Running in Place: Alternately jump with your left and right legs. The heel of the foot that remains on the ground is lifted slightly off the ground, not touching the floor. Increase the tempo until you run in place. Change directions while jumping.

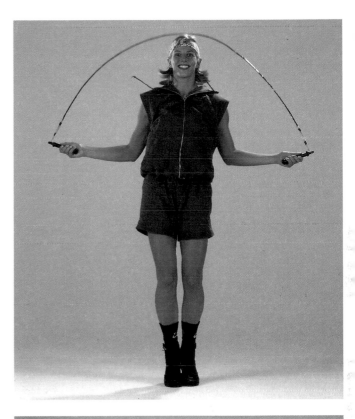

JUMPING ROPE 3

Double Jumps: This is the same exercise as # 2, but now you jump over the rope twice with the same foot. This exercise can be done at high speed. *It is important when jumping that your feet be only slightly off the floor.*

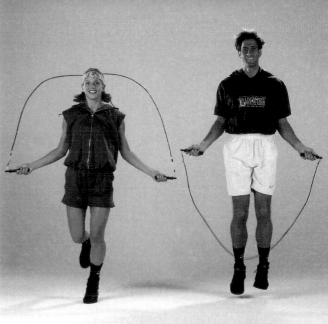

53

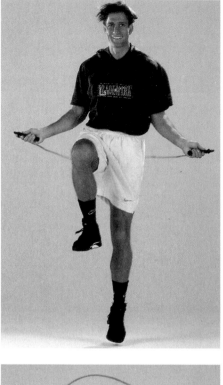

JUMPING ROPE 4

Knee-Lift Jumps: Alternately jump with your left and right legs, each time pulling your knee up high towards your body. After each one-leg jump, immediately use both legs when landing. Increase the intensity of the exercise by pulling your knees ever higher.

Variation:
   1. Do the same exercise, but without the intermediate jumps.

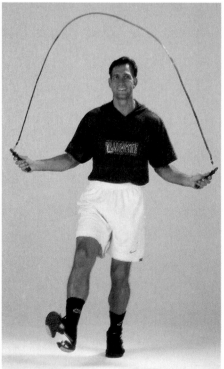

JUMPING ROPE 5

Kick Jumps: Jump alternately with your left and right legs while kicking the leg that is in the air forward. After each individual jump, do an intermediate jump with both legs.

Variation:
   1. Do the same exercise, but without the intermediate jumps.

JUMPING ROPE 6

Side Jumps: Alternately jump to the left and the right sides. Keep your legs together throughout and your feet parallel.

Variation:
1. Do the same exercise, but with intermediate jumps.

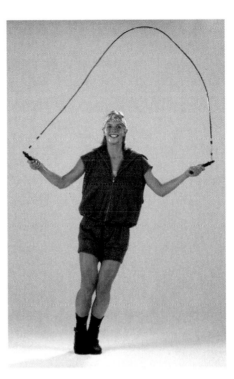

JUMPING ROPE 7

Step Jumps: Constantly alternate steps while jumping in place.

Variation:
1. Do the same exercises, but jump twice on each side.

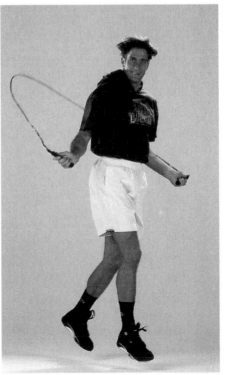

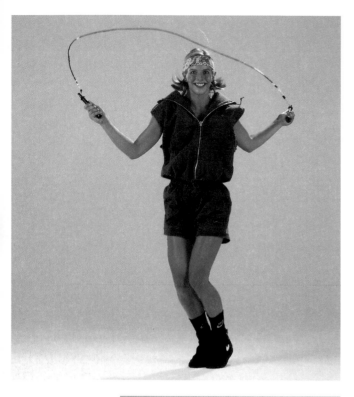

JUMPING ROPE 8

Twist Jumps: Twist your hips and both legs with every jump to the right and to the left. Keep your legs together throughout. Do an intermediate jump between each

Variation:
   1. Do the same exercise, but without intermediate jumps.

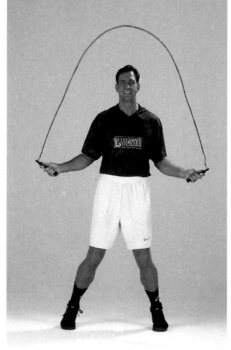

JUMPING ROPE 9

Jumping Jacks: Move your legs to the outside in the air during each jump and land on the floor in that position. Your knees should be slightly bent. Jump again and move your legs together, landing in that position (jumping jack).

JUMPING ROPE 10

Crossover Jumps: Do jumping jacks, but cross both legs alternatively in the air and land in each respective position. While crossing legs, alternate between the right leg in front of the left and the left in front of the right(see left, top photo).

JUMPING ROPE 11

Crossing Your Arms: While swinging the jump rope, cross your arms in front quickly and move them far enough to the outside so that you have room enough to jump through. Undo the crossover when the rope is behind your head and above your body. Continue with the basic jump(see right, top photo.)

JUMPING ROPE 12

Double Skips: Do a few basic jumps and increase your speed. Then pull your knees towards your body while jumping and quickly rotate the rope twice while you are still in the air. This is followed with an intermediate jump.

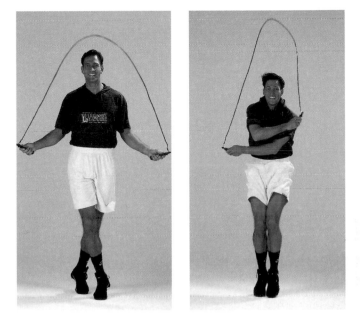

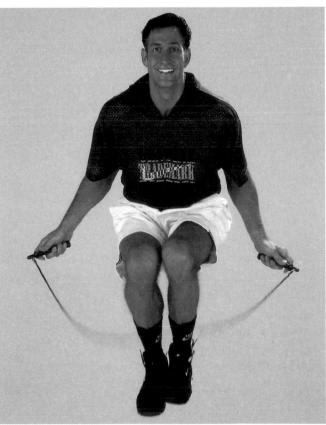

BOXING CIRCUIT

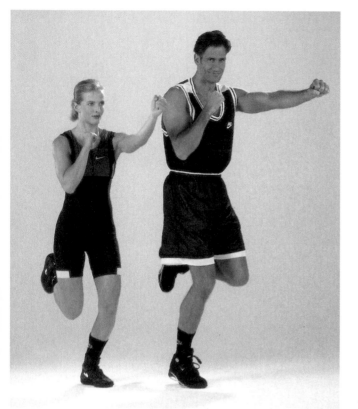

This type of workout uses different boxing-specific exercises. They are done consecutively in sequence. The duration and load of each individual exercise depends on your personal conditioning and the training program you have chosen. Each exercise is followed by a medium-to-short rest period.

BOXING CIRCUIT 1

Running in Place and Boxing: Run in place, holding your arms in their boxing positions. While running, alternately throw your fists forward. To increase the load, pull your knees up high while running or increase speed.

Variations:
   1. Alternately push your fists in the air while running in place.
   2. While running in place, kick your heels towards your buttocks.

BOXING CIRCUIT 2

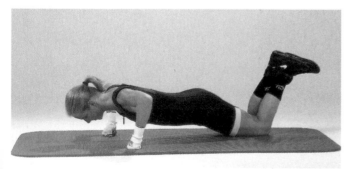

Push-Ups with Fists: Do push-ups using your fists as support. Your arms should be slightly bent and about shoulder-width apart. Keep your body muscles contracted and your body straight.
   Bend your elbows, lowering your body to the floor. Next, straighten your arms and assume the original

position. *It is important that you never straighten your elbows all the way and always keep your back straight.*

Variations:

1. Use your knees instead of feet as support. Cross the lower parts of your legs. Keep your body straight. This exercise is particularly good for untrained people or beginners (see the photo on the bottom of page 58).

2. Vary the position of your feet by keeping them close together, crossing them over, or setting them wide apart.

3. Vary the placement of your fists from close together to very far apart.

Variations:

1. Clasp your hands behind your head with your elbows pointing out.

2. Let your arms rest on each side of your body. Moving back into an upright position, bend your arms several times forward and up.

3. With your arms at your sides, bend them with each lunging step forward and straighten them when returning to an upright position (see the photo on this page).

4. Lift your arms to your sides at shoulder height. Move your arms either in front of your body or above your head each time you return to the set position.

BOXING CIRCUIT 3

Step-Knee Bends: Assume the set position. Lunge forward. Bend the knee of the leg that stepped forward, but not quite at right angles, and keep your foot flat on the floor. The knee of the rear leg should almost touch the floor. Return to your set position. *It is important that your back be straight and stretched.* Repeat this exercise phase several times and then change legs.

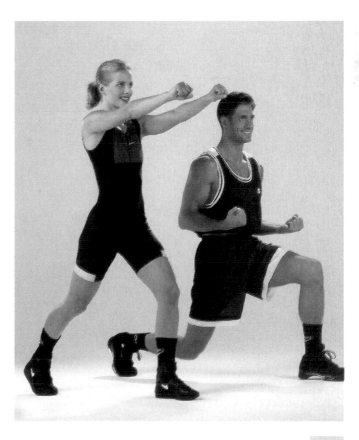

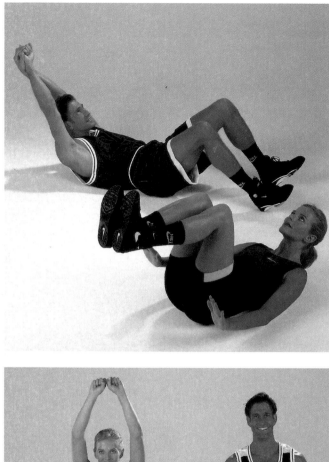

BOXING CIRCUIT 4

Crunches: Lying on your back, place your feet on the floor hip-distance apart. Push your heels against the floor and pull your toes up. Next, contract your stomach muscles and lift your shoulders off the floor. *It is important to keep your head straight.* From this position, lift your upper body up while pushing both hands forward. The lumbar region remains flat on the floor. Keep your chin up. Hold this position a few seconds, and then lower your back slowly to the floor.

Variations:
   1. Do the same exercise, but with your arms stretched above your head (see the left figure in the top photo).
   2. Do the same exercise, but move your hands alternately to the left and right of your knees.
   3. Do the same exercise, but cross your arms in front of your chest.
   4. Lift your feet off the floor, and bend your knees at right angles. Continue as described above with different variations (see the right figure in the top photo).

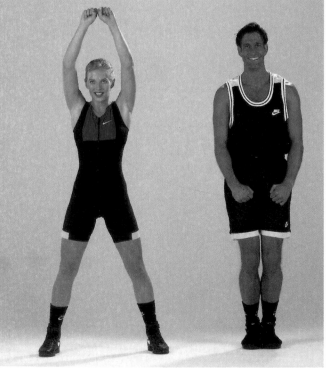

BOXING CIRCUIT 5

Jumping Jacks: Stand with your feet together (arms at your side) and then jump to a position with your legs spread and arms touching over your head. Return to your original position and continue as described.

BOXING CIRCUIT 6

Push-Up Jumps: Assume a prone position, supporting your body weight with your fists. Your arms should be almost straight. Bend one leg, with the foot as far forward as possible, until your knee is between both your arms. The other leg remains straight. Now, jump. Alternate between your left and right legs after each jump.

Variations:

1. Alternately jump with your legs to the side and back.

2. Jump forward and backward with both legs.

3. Do the same exercise as in 2, but when jumping back move both legs to the outside.

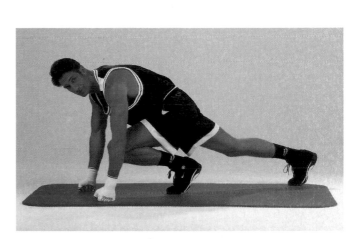

BOXING CIRCUIT 7

Knee Lifts to Elbow: Stand with your feet together, knees slightly bent. Clasp your hands behind your head with your elbows pointing out. Now, alternately lift your left and right knees high enough to touch the opposite elbow.

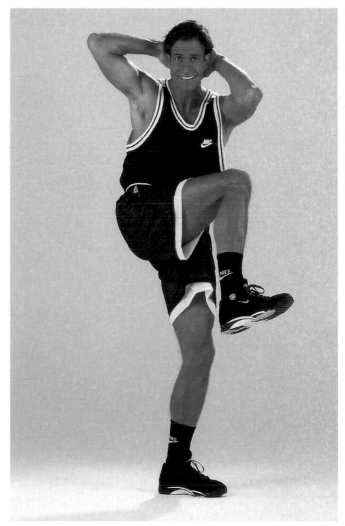

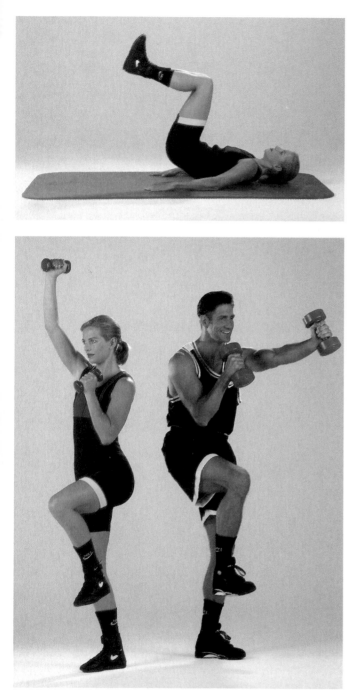

BOXING CIRCUIT 8

Pelvic Lifts: Lie on your back, and bend both your knees and hips at about right angles. Your arms should be on the floor next to your body with your palms on the floor. Flex your toes. Now, lift your pelvis off the floor, pressing your arms slightly against the floor for support. It is important that you do not pull your legs all the way up to your upper body; they should remain angled at your hip and knee joints.

Variations:
 1. Bend your elbows and place your arms at the sides of your head. The elbows should point out. Now, lift your pelvis.
 2. Lift your pelvis and lower your legs to the side until they rest on the floor. From this position, lift your pelvis again and return to the original position. Reverse sides.

BOXING CIRCUIT 9

Boxing with Heavy Hands: Hold a weight in each hand and assume the set position. Run in place and alternately push your fists forward.

Variation:
 1. Push both fists alternately upward.

BOXING CIRCUIT 10

Knee Bends and Neck Presses with Elastic Rope: Step on the rope with your feet about shoulder-width apart, and toes pointing out slightly. Hold the rope at its handles, and move your hands up to your head with your elbows bent at right angles. Now, contract your back muscles and bend your knees, keeping your heels flat on the floor. Push your arms and body up. *It is important that the elastic rope always be under tension.*

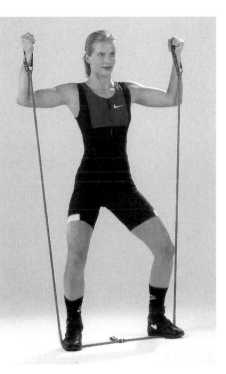

BOXING CIRCUIT 11

Crunches with Heavy Hands: Lying on your back, place your feet hip-distance apart as in Boxing Circuit 4. Hold the weights in your hands, lift your upper body off the floor, and push both arms forward.

Variations:

1. Do the same exercise, but lift the weights with bent arms to the temples of your head.

2. Do the same exercise, but lift your arms into defensive boxing positions and alternately push them out. You may want to pull your opposite knee up to your hand (see bottom photo).

3. Do the same exercise, but cross your arms in front of your chest.

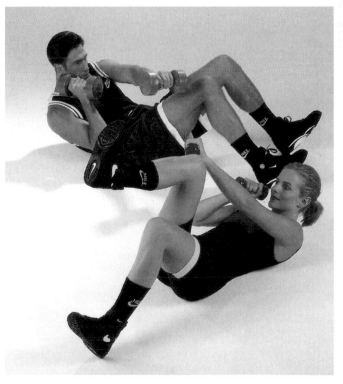

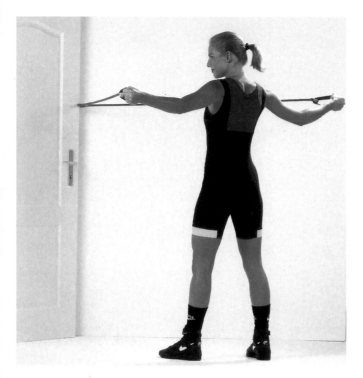

BOXING CIRCUIT 12

Elastic Rope for the Upper Back:
Secure the elastic rope to a sturdy surface, for instance, between a door frame and closed door. Place your hands into the loops. Lunge straight forward in the direction where the rope is anchored. Leave enough distance so that the elastic rope remains tense. Keep your upper body straight and slightly bent forward. Your arms should be almost perfectly straight and close to your body.

Push your elbows back and press your shoulder blades together. Make sure that all movements are carried out uniformly. Pull your arms forward, but stop before they are too close together.

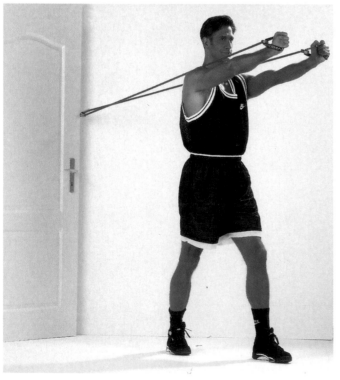

BOXING CIRCUIT 13

Elastic Rope for the Triceps: With the elastic rope securely fastened in the door frame and behind you, take one step forward and put your hands through the loops. Stand upright with your upper body bent slightly forward.

Bend your arms and lift your elbows up to shoulder level. Next, straighten both arms forward. Your elbows should remain at shoulder level.

PUNCHING

Since in real competition a boxer is fighting an opponent, it is important to simulate that situation during training. Focus mitts and heavy bags "substitute" for the opponent. When sparring is eliminated during fitness boxing, it is particularly important that alternative exercises with boxing equipment be available to exercise leg muscles, practice coordination, and develop a feel for distance and defensive positions (see also pages 27 to 36).

PUNCHING **1**

Straight Lefts to Speed Bag:
Assume a set position. Throw quick and easy jabs with your left hand, keeping your right hand in a defensive position. Straighten your arm when throwing the jab and pull back immediately for protection.

While throwing the jabs, slowly circle around the speed bag, or move closer to the speed bag or farther away. Pay attention to accurate distance. It should be far enough away so that your fist can just about reach the speed bag. It prevents the equipment from hitting you. *It is important to make sure that your defensive position is adequate.*

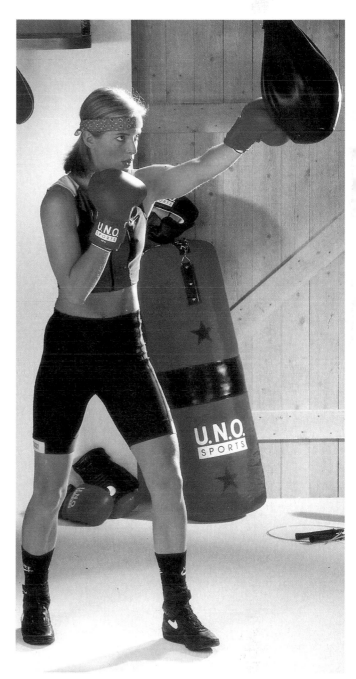

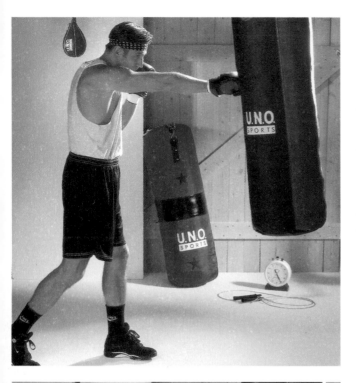

PUNCHING 2

Left/Right Jabs to the Heavy Bag:
Assume a set position. Then throw a straight left jab. Next, throw a right jab without reaching back. Pay attention to the rotation of your shoulder and hips, and make sure that the jabbing arm moves straight forward. Pull your arm back immediately after making impact and assume a defensive position. Put the whole weight of your body behind the punch to make it more powerful.

Variations:
  1. Vary the intensity of the punches.
  2. Punch and move about.

PUNCHING 3

Combination Punches: Assume the set position. In quick succession, throw a combination of different punches. Make sure that the combinations are thrown without pausing between the punches.

Variations:
  1. Alternately throw punches with your left and right hands.
  2. Throw two quick, light punches.
  3. Emphasize the right hand, which means a left jab followed by a short, hard right.
  4. Use explosive consecutive left-right-left punches. Speed here is important.
  5. Throw left-right-left punches and concentrate on one particular punch.

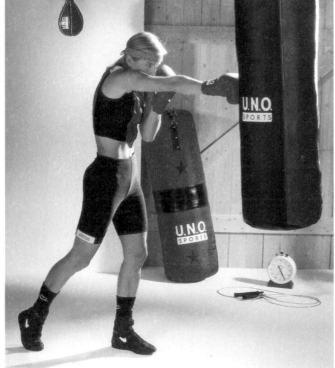

PUNCHING 4

Straight Rights with a Left Side Hook: Assume the set position. Use a quick, light straight jab followed immediately with a left side hook head-high. Immediately pull your arms back into defensive positions. Pay attention to the way your body rotates and concentrate on the hook. Take a short step while throwing a hook to reduce the distance and increase the power of your punch.

Variation:
  1. Throw side hooks to the body.

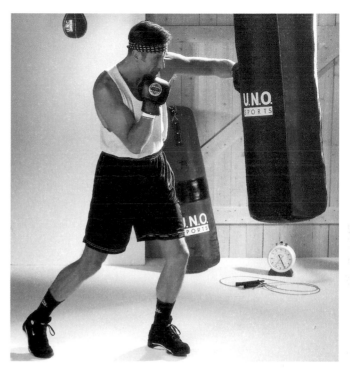

PUNCHING 5

Right Side Hooks: Assume a set position. With a quick left to the heavy bag, prepare for a head-high right side-hook. Shift your body weight to your left foot after impact (falling step); in this way, your whole body weight is put behind the punch. Your upper body should slightly bend to the left because during competition you must duck away from the opponent's straight counterpunch. If that should be the case, your left hand will block the hitting hand of the opponent.

Variation:
  1. Throw a left head-high (where the opponent is protected) and use your right for a side hook to the body.

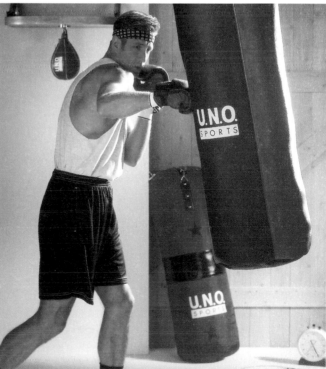

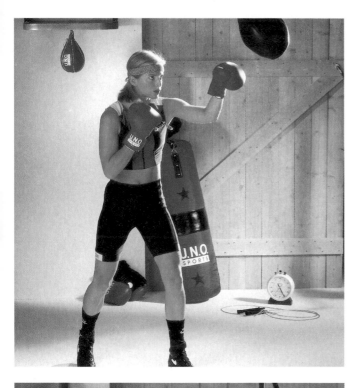

PUNCHING 6

Running in Place and Hitting the Speed Bag: Assume a set position. Using quick, lengthened, straight-forward lefts, drive your fists into the speed bag while running in place with short steps. Then step back as you throw two straight left punches *(attention: the speed bag bounces back quickly)* and stop the speed bag with a powerful punch with your right. Keep your proper distance and move back quickly.

PUNCHING 7

Combinations to the Speed Bag: Assume a set position. Hit the speed bag with a series of different hooks. Because the speed bag bounces back quickly and constantly, this exercise is also a good training to practice avoidance movements.

Variations:
    1. Use a straight-straight-straight combination.
    2. Use a straight-hook-straight combination.
    3. Use a straight-hook-hook combination.
    4. Use a hook-hook-hook combination.

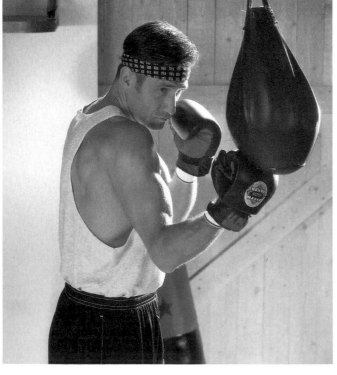

PUNCHING 8

Left/Right Uppercuts: Assume a set position. Then throw left/right uppercuts to where the opponent's head or body would be. Later, combine these punches with side hooks and straight jabs.

Variations:

    1. Throw uppercuts, a side hook, and another side hook.
    2. Throw a side hook, another side hook, and an uppercut.
    3. Throw an uppercut, a straight jab, and another straight jab.
    4. Throw a straight jab, a side hook, and an uppercut.

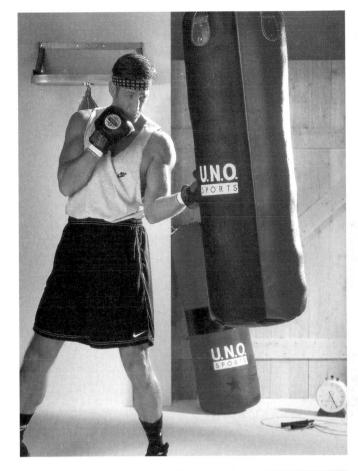

PUNCHING 9

Practicing Speed Punching: Assume a set position. Now, alternately throw left/right jabs without pausing in between. What is important here is speed, not technically correct execution. Each set is followed by a rest period. The duration of the rest period should be the same as the exercise period; for instance, 10 seconds of rest for 10 seconds of exercise, 15 seconds for 15 seconds, 30 seconds for 30 seconds, etc., depending on the person's conditioning.

Variations:

    1. Throw only successive straight left jabs.
    2. Throw only successive straight right jabs.

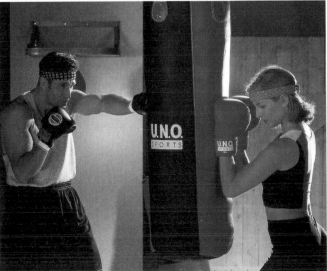

TRAINING WITH A PARTNER

Exercising with a partner is a very important part of a boxing workout. It is an easy way to learn specific offensive and defensive techniques and a good way to practice the use of focus mitts. In fitness boxing, sparring is eliminated.

What follows is an introduction to a workout with focus mitts. The partner who is holding the padded gloves is in a unique position to observe, control, and correct the hitting actions of the other because he/she sees the action from the point of view of an opponent. Another advantage is that working with a partner simulates boxing movements, which provides legwork. In addition, it is a chance to get a feeling for distance, and provides exercise for all the muscles in your body.

The way the focus mitts are held and moved around determines the direction and technique of the punching. In this way, a constant switch from offensive to defensive actions is taking place.

Working with a partner with focus mitts is very strenuous and very intense, and movements come very close to actual competitive fights. However, what is missing are the psychological components of boxing competition or sparring, which can be extreme that occur when the opponent hits back.

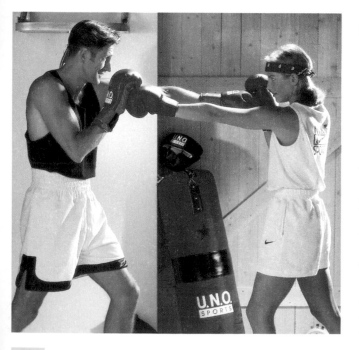

PARTNER TRAINING 1

Hitting/Protecting: Assume a set position and practice the following hitting and defensive combinations:

Variations:
1. You and your partner should alternately throw a straight left jab to the chin and deflect the other's punch with your right fist in front of your chin (see photo).
2. Do the same exercise described in # 1, but instead of a left jab throw a straight right jab, which is deflected with the left hand.
3. Your partner should throw a straight left jab to your body. Defend against the hit with your right elbow and counter with a left straight to

the chin of your partner who, in turn, will deflect this action with his right fist.

4. Your partner should make a straight left jab in the direction of your head. You deflect his left to the left with your right fist while moving slightly forward to the right. Now, use your left hand to make a straight jab to the body of your partner, who, in turn, will deflect this with his right fist to the outside (see top photo).

5. Do the same exercise described in # 4, but instead of a straight left jab throw an uppercut.

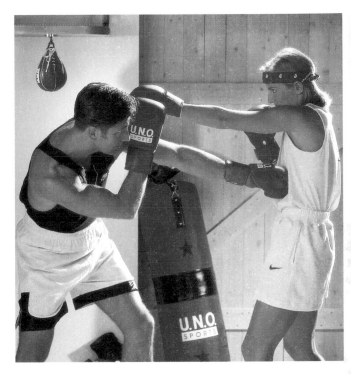

PARTNER TRAINING 2

Ducking and Weaving: Use the avoidance and evasive movements discussed on page 35. Do these movements with a partner.

PARTNER TRAINING 3

Sudden Lefts/Rights While Moving: Assume a set position opposite your partner and full distance from him/her. As soon as your partner lifts a left focus mitt, throw a left jab at the center of the mitt with lightning speed. It is important that you hit quickly and accurately.

Variations:

1. Do the same exercise, but throw a straight left instead (see photo on bottom).

2. Do the same exercise while moving.

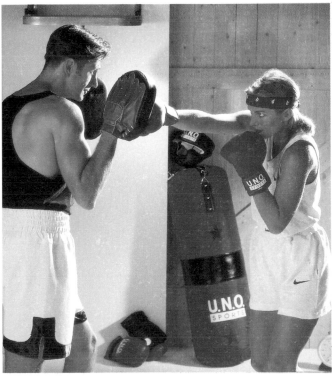

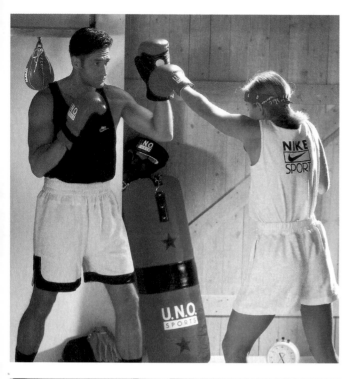

PARTNER TRAINING 4

Single and Double Jabs: Assume a set position opposite your partner. Throw a left jab while moving. Move in small steps and change directions. Hit with lightning speed from a protective position and immediately pull back in a defensive position.

Variations:
   1. Throw two quick jabs in succession.
   2. Throw alternately with your left and right hands.

PARTNER TRAINING 5

Side Hooks: Your partner holds the focus mitt slightly turned so that your fist hits the mitt straight-on with a hook. Hit the focus mitt diagonally from the opposite side.

Variation:
   1. Prepare for your hit with a straight jab.

PARTNER TRAINING 6

Uppercuts: Your partner holds the focus mitt in front of his body, angled slightly down. Depending on the position of the focus mitt, you can now throw an uppercut to the body or head. *It is important to hit accurately from a defensive position.*

Variation:
   1. Prepare for the uppercut with a straight jab.

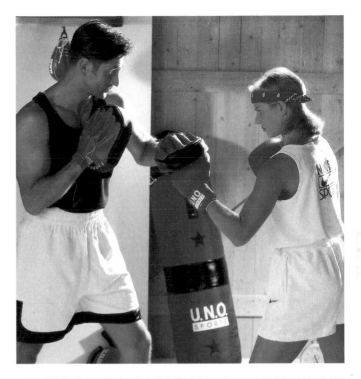

PARTNER TRAINING 7

Moving Back/Left-Left-Right Combinations: Assume a set position. Your partner should move towards you. Move back and throw a straight jab with your left twice, which forces your partner into a defensive position. Now, suddenly stand still, with a solid stance, and with lightning speed hit the focus mitt with a straight right jab.

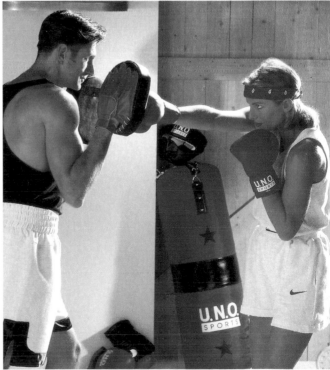

COOLDOWN

Your fitness-boxing exercises have tired your body considerably. Cooldown exercises at the conclusion of your workout help your body recuperate. To cool down, choose dynamic exercises that decrease in intensity and involve as many muscle groups as possible while, at the same time, they slowly lower your pulse rate.

Stretching exercises are particularly important during the cooldown phase. They loosen your muscles and dissolve minor cramps. Stretching your muscles slowly and holding this stretch for at least 20 seconds are the most effective ways of stretching.

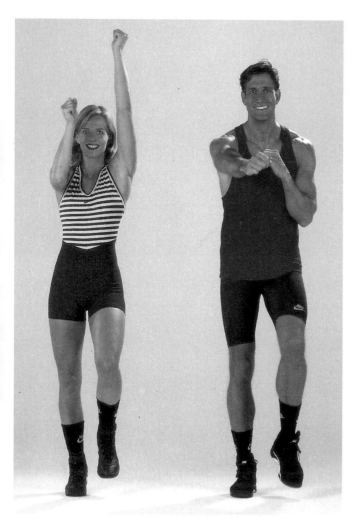

COOLDOWN **1**

Running in Place While Boxing:
Gently run in place with your arms at all times in their defensive position in front of your upper body. Relax and alternately throw left/right straight jabs. You can also throw your fists up or down. Use one minute each for punching forward, up and down, and forward again.

Cooldown 2

Relaxed Jump Kicks with Arm Lifts:
In relaxed fashion, jump in place while kicking your legs to the sides and forward. After one intermediate jump, land on both feet before jumping with the other leg. During the jumps, move your arms from the center of your body to your sides and up to shoulder height.

Cooldown 3

Running in Place with Ice-Skating Steps: With your upper body bent slightly forward, take gliding ice-skating steps. With every step to the outside, move your other leg also in the direction of the glide. Your arms can swing rhythmically forward and back or simply move very relaxed along the side of your body (see bottom left photo).

Cooldown 4

Side to Side with Your Arms:
Assume the final stance. Spread your legs more than shoulder-width apart and rotate your knees, which are slightly bent, to the outside. Now, alternately shift your body weight from left to right and support your body as it stretches by moving the opposite arm up above your head (see bottom right photo).

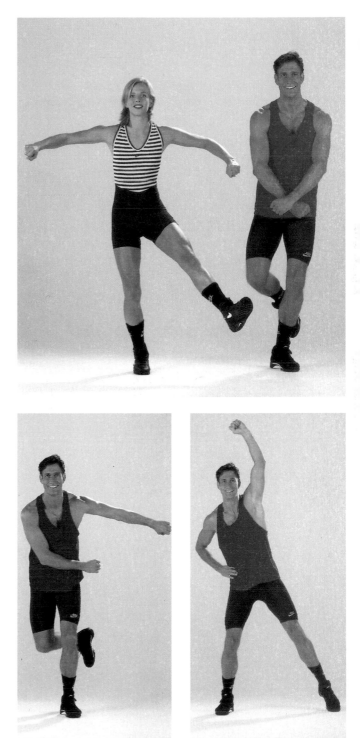

STRETCHING

When you stretch your muscles, you keep them taut for a short period. During the warm-up exercises, muscles are tensed for about 30 seconds, and during cooldown for at least 20 seconds.

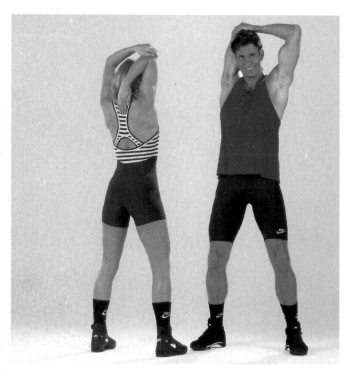

STRETCHING 1

Stretching Your Arm Muscles: Stand upright with your knees and hips slightly bent. Your feet should be approximately shoulder-width apart. Move one hand behind your head to your upper back between the shoulder blades. With your other hand, hold and pull on your elbow. Switch sides.

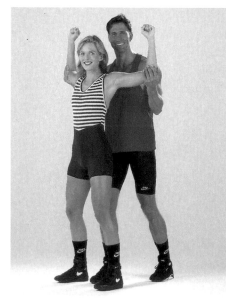

STRETCHING 2

Stretching Your Chest Muscles: Stand in front of your partner with your back facing him, arms slightly bent. Lift your arms to shoulder height. Your partner now holds your elbows and pulls your arms back with even pressure. Keep your chest and stomach muscles contracted.

STRETCHING 3

Stretching Your Shoulder Blades:
Assume a final stance. Your knees
and hips should be slightly bent, and
your feet should be hip-distance
apart. Lace your fingers and raise
your arms chest- high with your
palms forward. Now, push both your
arms slowly as far forward as
possible. This pulls your shoulder
blades apart and makes your back
slightly rounded.

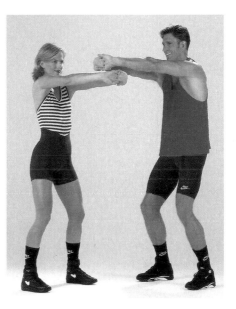

STRETCHING 4

Stretching Your Hip Flexor: Assume
a forward-lunging step. Place your
rear leg as far back as possible.
Now, push your pelvis forward while
keeping your back straight.

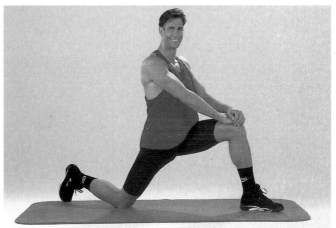

STRETCHING 5

**Stretching Your Thigh and Buttock
Muscles:** Lie on your back. Grab one
leg behind the knee with both of your
hands and pull your thigh as close to
your chest as possible. Straighten
your leg slowly and pull your toes
towards your body.*The muscles of
the leg on the floor should remain
contracted.*

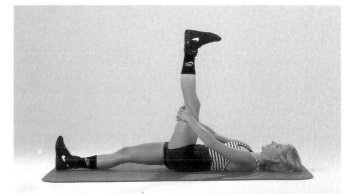

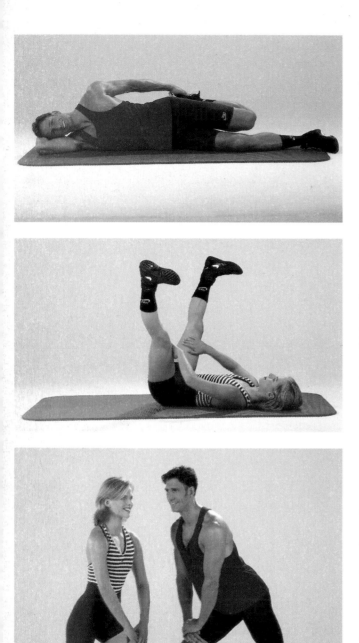

STRETCHING 6

Leg Pulls: This exercise stretches the front of the thigh muscles and front of the lower leg muscles. Do the following: Lie down on one side. Reach for your toes and pull your heel towards your buttocks. Your knees should remain parallel to each other. Stabilize your pelvis by contracting your stomach and buttock muscles.

STRETCHING 7

Leg Spreads: This exercise stretches the muscles at the insides of the legs. Do the following: Lie down on your back. Lift your legs and stretch them towards the ceiling while spreading them apart as far apart as possible. Place your hands on the inside of your thighs to increase the stretch, and pull the tips of your toes actively towards your body.

STRETCHING 8

Standing Steps: This exercise stretches the calf muscles. Do the following: Assume a lunging position. Shift your body weight to your front leg. Your toes should point forward and your heel should not be raised off the floor. Now, push your hips forward without raising your heel off the floor. The lower you bend your forward leg, the more effective the stretching will be on the calf muscles of your rear leg.

SPECIFIC TRAINING PROGRAMS

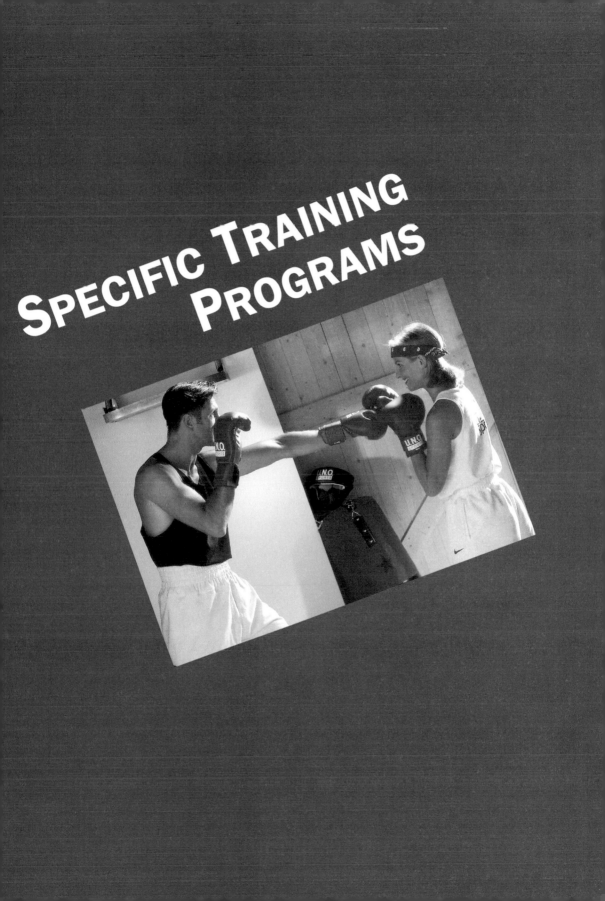

DESIGN OF A TRAINING UNIT

Each training unit (TU) is organized according to the following schedule:

Phase	Content	Duration
1	Warm-up exercises	at least 10 minutes
2	**Boxing training program**	depending on the program
	Aerobic boxing and/or jumping rope	5–10 minutes
	Punching	5–10 minutes
	Partner Training	5–20 minutes
	Boxing Circuit	5–15 minutes
3	Cooldown, Stretching	5–10 minutes
After TU	Regeneration (relaxing, massage, etc.)	as long as you like

A warm-up is designed to prepare the body for exercise by raising your pulse rate and to minimize the danger of injuries. Warm-up exercises done with increasing intensity stimulate the circulatory system, breathing, and metabolism and stretch muscles. At the same time, the warm-up is a mental preparation for the workout that is to follow. After this fine-tuning you may choose any one of the suggested boxing training programs that follow, keeping in mind your individual goals and capabilities.

The cooldown exercises at the conclusion of a workout prepare the body for the recovery phase. This is the most important phase for a successful training program because exercising makes you tired, which temporarily weakens the body, and this phase allows you to recover. The stretching exercises in the cooldown phase are particularly important because they lengthen muscles that have worked hard. They serve to keep the muscles supple and the joints functioning properly.

Since the body's answers to an increased exercise load is exhaustion, allow a sufficient amount of time to recuperate (see the photo below). Therefore, the next phase is recovery. The amount of time needed for recovery depends on the type of workout and how well a person is conditioned. For the training programs described here, we recommend that for boxing, the beginner and the advanced athlete allow 48 hours (two days) for recovery. For the more intense power programs, a recovery period of three days is necessary.

The recovery phase can be optimized if you combine it with relaxing activities, such as sitting or lying down, going to a sauna, taking a warm bath, and if you supplement your nutrition with high-quality vitamins, carbohydrates, and mineral-rich food and drinks. During the recovery period, the depleted energy reservoir, for a short period of time, can be replenished beyond the level that existed at the beginning of the exercises. This is called super-compensation. If you use this level of energy as a new stimulus for your training, you will accomplish the greatest possible increase in your performance (see chart on page 82).

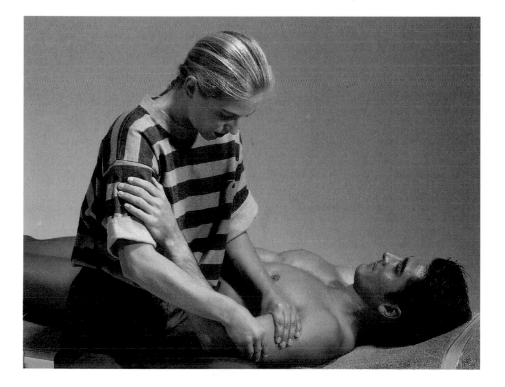

LONG-TERM TRAINING

Any fitness program can only give you the desired results if it is implemented regularly. This also holds for fitness boxing. The way your training program is designed depends on your individual, realistic capabilities. Beginners and untrained athletes should choose a program that is less intense and is not too long and, during the initial phases, has only a few boxing-specific exercises.

The body needs two weeks to adjust to this new level of activity. For that reason, for the first two weeks engage in aerobic boxing, jumping rope, and the boxing circuit as well as the warm-up and cooldown exercises. Training programs #1 and #2, boxing for beginners and advanced athletes, are particularly useful in this instance. Later, slowly increase the load and the duration of your workouts, always alternating between programs. Expand your programs to exercising with equipment (punching on the heavy bag and speed bag) and partner-training (working with focus mitts). (See programs 3 to 7.)

Since your joints and ligaments need to adjust to the new training load, take these suggestions seriously. Those who have been involved in a regular fitness program can start with boxing-specific exercise programs, because they have already built the foundation.

If you follow the proper guidelines while training and recuperating, it will lead to an increased level of performance in the next training phase. This is called super-compensation.

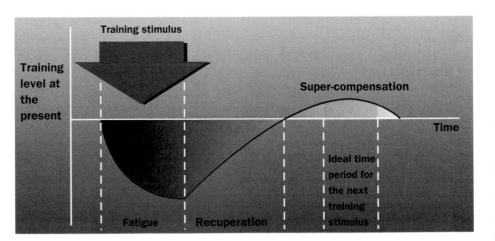

TRAINING PROGRAMS

Depending on your capabilities and training goals, choose from the following training programs:

- ❖ **Boxing for Beginners**

- ❖ **Boxing for the Advanced**

- ❖ **Boxing for Professionals**
  Geared to Boxing Competition

- ❖ **Super-conditioning**
  for Stamina

- ❖ **Technique/Power**
  for Boxing Techniques

- ❖ **Power Circuit**
  for Stamina

- ❖ **Pace and Power**
  for Speed and Power

No matter which program you choose, it is imperative that you warm up sufficiently before you start. We recommend the exercises from the warm-up and stretching programs (on pages 44 to 46 and 76 to 78). The warm-up exercises should take about 10 minutes and gradually prepare the body for the workout.

After the warm up, you may begin with any one of the training programs. Beginners should start with program #1 and later advance to #2. Those who are more advanced and already have some experience with boxing workouts can choose programs # 3 and 5, particularly if boxing-specific training is the goal. Programs #4, 6, and 7 are designed to address conditioning, that is, stamina, power and speed.

The training programs are designed with elements from different exercise units. Their exercises were chosen according to how they improve stamina, power, or coordination.

When starting a training program, begin with aerobic boxing and rope-jumping exercises. These can then be followed by punching exercises and partner-training. The exercises listed in the section Boxing Circuit all work well as the conclusion of a training session.

Exercises in the circuit program are designed so that each exercise is done, in the case of beginners or advanced athletes, for 20 or 30 seconds. A short rest period of 15 to 20 seconds follows before you continue with the next exercise.

Every training session should be concluded with a cooldown which includes relaxation and stretching exercises.

Note: A number appears before each exercise. This number refers to the designation of that exercise as it was described in a previous chapter.

Program 1: Boxing for Beginners

Aerobic Boxing (pages 47 to 51)
▶ Approximately 20 seconds, continuously for several rounds

1 Step-touch boxing
2 Heel-touch boxing
3 Step-jump boxing
4 Squat boxing
5 Knee lifts with arms

Training with a Partner (pages 70 to 73)
▶ Do each exercise for two minutes.
▶ Partners should change positions every 30 seconds.
▶ If no partner is available, shadow box (using different hits and combinations) in 2-minute increments in front of the mirror.

1 Hitting/protecting
2 Ducking and weaving
3 Sudden lefts/rights while moving

Jumping Rope (pages 52 to 57)
▶ Every 30 seconds, change exercises (5 minutes total)

1 Basic jumps
2 Running in place while jumping rope

Punching (pages 65 to 69)
▶ One round of two minutes each, one minute rest:

1 Straight lefts to speed bag
2 Left/right jabs to the heavy bag

Boxing Circuit (pages 58 to 64)
▶ 20 seconds with 20-second rest period in between.

1 Running in place while boxing
2 Push-ups with fists
3 Step-knee bends
4 Crunches
7 Knee lifts to elbow

Aerobic Boxing (pages 47 to 51)

▶ Approximately 20 to 30 seconds consecutively during several rounds.

1 Step-touch boxing

3 Step-jump boxing

4 Squat boxing

6 Boxing step forward/backwards

7 Falling steps different combos

9 Back-and-forth ducking

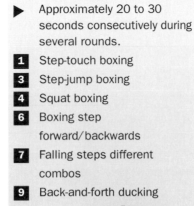

Training with a Partner (pages 70 to 73)

▶ Do each exercise for 2 minutes

▶ Partners should change positions every 30 seconds

▶ If no partner is available, shadow box (using different punches and combinations) in 2-minute increments in front of the mirror.

1 Hitting/protecting (variations)

2 Ducking and weaving

4 Single and double jabs

5 Side hooks

Jumping Rope (pages 52 to 57)

▶ Every 30 seconds change exercise (for a total of 7-10 minutes).

1 Basic jumps

4 Knee-lift jumps

5 Kick jumps

6 Side jumps

Punching (pages 65 to 69)

▶ One round each for two minutes, and one-minute rest.

2 Left/right jabs to heavy bag

3 Combination exercises to the heavy bag

4 Straight rights with left side hooks to heavy bag

7 Combinations to speed bag

Boxing Circuit (pages 58 to 64)

▶ 20 to 30 seconds with 15 to 20 seconds rest.

1 Running in place and boxing

2 Push-ups with fists

3 Step-knee bends

4 Crunches (variations)

6 Push-up jumps

7 Knee lifts to elbows

9 Boxing with Heavy Hands

Aerobic Boxing (pages 47 to 51)

▶ 30 seconds for each exercise. Do these exercises several times.

1 Step-touch boxing
2 Heel-touch boxing
5 Knee lifts with arms
6 Boxing steps forward/backward
7 Falling steps (variations)
8 Side-lunge boxing
9 Back-and-forth ducking

Jumping Rope (pages 52 to 57)

▶ Every 30 seconds change exercises (for a total of 10 minutes).

2 Running in place
3 Double jumps
4 Knee-lift jumps
6 Side jumps
8 Twist jumps
9 Jumping jacks
11 Crossing your arms

Punching (pages 65 to 69)

▶ Three minutes each exercise, one-minute rest period.

2 Left/right jabs to the heavy bag
3 Combination exercises to the heavy bag
6 Running in place and hitting the speed bag
7 Combinations to speed bag
9 Speed punching

Training with a Partner (pages 70 to 73)

▶ Two minutes each exercise.
▶ Partners should change positions every 30 seconds.
▶ Should no partner be available, shadow box (using different punches and combinations) two to three minutes in front of the mirror.

1 Hitting/protecting)
2 Ducking and weaving
3 Sudden left/right jabs while moving
4 Single and double jabs
5 Side hooks
6 Uppercuts

Boxing Circuit (pages 58 to 64)

▶ 30 seconds each exercise, with 15 seconds rest in between.

1 Running in place and boxing
2 Push-ups with fists
3 Step-knee bends
4 Crunches (Variations)
5 Jumping jacks
6 Push-up jumps
8 Pelvic lifts
12 Elastic rope for upper back
13 Elastic rope for triceps

Boxing Circuit (pages 58 to 64)

► 30 seconds with high intensity, then 15-second pause, then change exercises (3 rounds).

► Depending on level of training, shorten pauses.

► Pauses should, on average, be 3 minutes.

1. Running in place while boxing
2. Push-ups with fists
3. Step-knee bends
4. Crunches (variations)
5. Jumping jacks
6. Push-up jumps
7. Knee-lifts to elbow
8. Pelvic lifts
9. Boxing with Heavy Hands
10. Knee bends and neck presses with elastic rope
11. Crunches with weights
12. Elastic rope for the upper back
13. Elastic rope for the triceps

Jumping Rope (pages 52 to 57)

► Every 30 seconds, change exercises(for a total of 10 minutes) after warming up 5 to 10 minutes.

1. Basic jumps
2. Running in place
3. Double jumps
4. Knee-lift jumps
5. Kick jumps
6. Side jumps
7. Step jumps
9. Jumping jacks
10. Crossover jumps
11. Crossing your arms
12. Double skips

Punching (pages 65 to 69)

► One round 3 minutes each, 1-minute pause.

3. Combinations to the heavy bag
6. Running in place and hitting the speed bag
7. Speed bag combinations
9. Speed punching

Aerobic Boxing (pages 47 to 51)

▶ Approximately 20 seconds, continuously for several rounds

2 Heel-touch boxing

3 Step-jump boxing (variations)

6 Boxing steps forwards and backward

8 Side-lunge boxing

Training with a Partner (pages 70 to 73)

▶ Do each exercise for 2 minutes.

▶ Partners should change position every 30 seconds.

▶ When no partner is available, **shadow box** (with different punches and combinations) two to three minutes in front of a mirror.

4 Single and double jabs

7 Moving back/ left-left-right combinations

As an option, shadow boxing

Jumping Rope (pages 52 to 57)

▶ Change exercises, every 30 seconds (total of 5 to 10 minutes).

6 Side jumps

7 Step jumps

8 Twist jumps

9 Jumping jacks

10 Crossover jumps

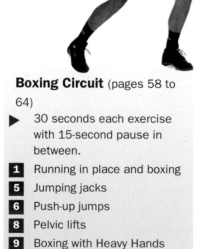

Punching (pages 65 to 69)

▶ Each round three minutes, one-minute pause. Box 2 to 3 rounds, concluding with exercise #9.

3 Combinations to heavy bag

6 Running in place and hitting the speed bag

7 Combinations to speed bag

9 Speed punches

Boxing Circuit (pages 58 to 64)

▶ 30 seconds each exercise with 15-second pause in between.

1 Running in place and boxing

5 Jumping jacks

6 Push-up jumps

8 Pelvic lifts

9 Boxing with Heavy Hands

Aerobic Boxing (pages 47 to 51)
- ▶ 30 seconds consecutively, three rounds.
- **2** Heel-touch boxing
- **6** Boxing steps forwards/backward
- **7** Falling steps (variations)
- **9** Back-and-forth ducking

Training with a Partner
(pages 70 to 73)
- ▶ Each exercise for 2 minutes.
- ▶ Partners should change positions every 30 seconds.
- ▶ When no partner is available, **shadow box** (with the use of different punches and combinations) 2 to 3 minutes in front of a mirror.
- **1** Hitting/protecting (variations)
- **2** Ducking and weaving
- **3** Sudden lefts/rights while moving
- **4** Single and double jabs
- **5** Side hooks
- **6** Uppercuts
- **7** Pulling back/left-left-right combinations

Jumping Rope (pages 52 to 57)
- ▶ Change exercises every 30 seconds (total of 5 to 10 minutes
- **2** Running in place
- **3** Double jumps
- **8** Twist jumps
- **9** Jumping jacks
- **11** Crossing your arms

Punching (pages 65 to 69)
- ▶ Each round three minutes, one-minute pause.
- **4** Straight rights with left side hooks to the heavy bag
- **5** Right side hooks to the heavy bag
- **7** Combinations to speed bag
- **8** Left/right uppercuts to the heavy bag

Boxing Circuit
(pages 58 to 64)
- ▶ 30 seconds, 15-second pause.
- **6** Push-up jumps
- **7** Knee lifts to elbow
- **8** Pelvic lifts
- **10** Knee bends and neck presses with elastic rope

Aerobic Boxing (pages 47 to 51)

▶ 30 seconds each, consecutively for three rounds.

3 Step–jump boxing
4 Squat boxing
8 Side-lunge boxing

Training with a Partner (pages 70 to 73)

▶ Each exercise 2 minutes. Partners should change positions every 30 seconds.

▶ If no partner is available, **shadow box** (using different punches and combinations) two to three minutes in front of the mirror.

3 Sudden left/rights while moving
5 Side hooks

Jumping Rope (pages 52 to 57)

▶ Change exercises every 30 seconds (total of 10 minutes).

4 Knee-lift jumps
6 Side jumps
8 Twist jumps
12 Double skips

Boxing Circuit (pages 58 to 64)

30 seconds with 15-second pause.

5 Jumping jacks
8 Pelvic lifts
9 Boxing with Heavy Hands
10 Knee bends and neck presses with elastic rope
11 Crunches with weights
12 Elastic rope for the upper back
13 Elastic rope for the triceps

Punching (pages 65 to 69)

▶ Each round three minutes, one-minute pause.

▶ Box 2 to 3 rounds, concluding with exercise #9.

2 Left/right jabs to the heavy bag
3 Combinations to heavy bag
7 Combinations to speed bag
9 Speed punches

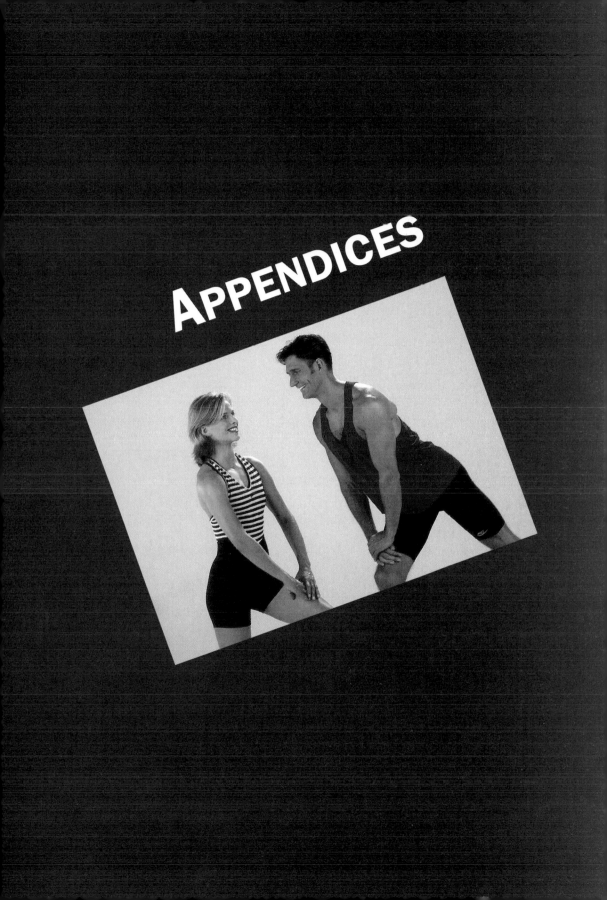

APPENDICES

GLOSSARY

Aerobic Boxing Specific exercises that have boxing and aerobic elements.

Avoidance Movement A boxing technique in which the upper body moves back.

Basic Left Stance The position a right-handed boxer takes. The left hand is the leading hand, and the right the punching hand.

Basic Right Stance The position a left-handed boxer takes. The right hand is the leading hand, and the left hand is the hitting hand.

Boxing Boots Light, medium-high athletic shoes with little or no cushion.

Boxing Gloves Leather mittens heavily padded on their backs which are used for sparring and boxing.

Brawler A boxer more interested in power-hitting than in boxing technique.

Circuit A type of training in which several exercises are carried out consecutively.

Cross Punch A counterpunch to the head, usually with the hitting hand. This punch moves above the leading hand of the opponent.

Crunch An exercise that is used to strengthen the stomach muscles.

Defensive Posture A position or posture where the punches of the opponent are deflected with the arms, fists, or shoulder so that they are rendered ineffective (no points are earned by the opponent).

Distance The distance between the boxer and his opponent, allowing for the full use of his arm.

Diving An avoidance movement caused by bending one's knees.

Double Defense A boxing tactic in which both arms protect the body. Either both shield the head or the body, or one arm shields the body, and one the head.

Elastic Bandage A bandage used as protection for finger and hand joints and to stabilize the wrist.

Elastic Rope A tube-shaped rope with handles on each end that creates resistance when pulled, thereby strengthening the muscles that are engaged.

Focus Mitts Gloves with oval-shaped leather cushions on their backs. They serve as a target for practicing hitting accuracy, coordination, and different combinations.

Half Distance The distance at which the opponent is close enough so that a straight jab and a hook can be thrown.

Heavy Bag A training bag used to practice punching. It substitutes for an actual opponent.

Hitting combination A combination of at least two different basic hits.

Hitting Hand The hand held close to the body. It has more hitting power than the leading hand.

Hook A classic punch to the head or body that is speeded up when the body is twisted. It is the most frequently used punch in boxing.

Infight A situation in which boxers fight body-to-body and throw hooks.

Jab. Quick punches with the leading hand, thrown constantly to keep the opponent engaged and at a distance.

Jump Rope A hemp, rubber, or steel rope used for warming up and to improve conditioning.

Knockout The termination of a boxing match in which one boxer has been knocked down and is unable to rise and resume boxing within a ten count.

Leading Hand The hand that keeps the opponent at a distance and also prepares for offensive tactics.

Light Gloves Gloves used when exercising with boxing equipment. These gloves have minimum padding.

Low Blow Hitting below the belt.

Parry Deflecting or pushing an opponent's punch away.

Punch A hard hit in boxing.

Punching Bag A stuffed or inflated bag that is suspended for free movement and is punched for exercise or training.

Shuffle To move back and forth in the boxing ring.

Side Roll Rolling the upper body to the side.

Side Step An avoidance movement with quick, flat steps and slight body rotation.

Sparring Training with a boxing partner in a way that resembles an actual competition fight.

Speed Bag A pear-shaped leather bag filled with corn used to practice punching. It extends from the ceiling at head height.

Straight Punch An offensive punch in which the arm moves forward in a straight line.

Technical Knockout The termination of a fight by the referee because of an injury or because he fears the opponent is in danger.

Uppercut A powerful hook thrown from below to the chin or head.

Weaving An avoidance movement in which the upper body of the boxer turns to the side.

Photo Credits: Page 9—AKG, Berlin; all other photos—STUDIO TEAM Gesellschaft für Werbefotografie mbH/W. Zöltsch, Langen.

INDEX